I0412550

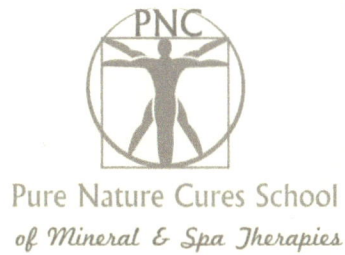

Pure Nature Cures School
of Mineral & Spa Therapies

How Clays Work

Science and Applications of Clays and Clay-like Minerals in Health & Beauty

Galina St George

All Rights Reserved. No part of this publication may be reproduced in any form or by any means, including scanning, photocopying, or otherwise without prior written permission of the copyright holder.
Copyright © 2020

Table of Contents

1. Disclaimer

The author of this book sincerely believes that a natural approach to health and maintaining a natural balance within the human body are very important in experiencing energy, vitality, and vibrant health throughout life.

The author recognizes that opinions within scientific and medical fields differ greatly. The purpose of this book is to share educational information and scientific research gathered as a result of years of research by the author, scientists, and informed advocates of health and well-being using natural methods and resources.

None of the information contained in this book is intended to diagnose, prevent, treat, or cure any disease, nor is it intended to prescribe any of the techniques, materials or concepts presented as a form of treatment for any illness or medical condition.

Before beginning any practice pertaining to procedures described in the book, it is highly recommended that you first obtain the consent and advice of a licensed health care professional.

The author assumes no responsibility for the choices you make after you review the information contained herein and your consultation with a licensed healthcare professional.

While the author of this book does everything possible to provide valid reference sources of the information cited in this book it is important to remember that unlike printed materials, online content is constantly changing. For this reason, some of the web references provided in the book may have expired due to such changes and become invalid at the time of reading. The author bears no responsibility for these changes and invalidation of the reference sources.

2. Introduction

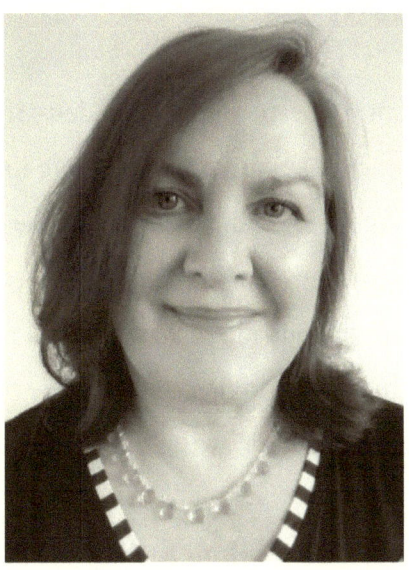

Natural health practitioners believe that the body has all the necessary resources to heal itself. Nature has provided for it generously, both within and out. Clays are perhaps some of the most ancient remedies used by people and animals to accelerate healing.

Clays work in gentle, intuitive ways, by re-tuning the body systems and stimulating recovery. This is not to say that medicines should be abandoned in favour of clays. This is merely to say that clays have a well-deserved place in our health and beauty routines.

I use clays regularly myself - both internally (drinking clay water) and externally (baths, compresses, body washes).

The most important property of clay is to detoxify the body, due to its ability to attract positively-charged toxic ions (clay particles are negatively charged) and take them out of the body. A lot of our illnesses happen due to contamination of the body with toxins – both coming from the outside (environmental pollutants), and produced inside (metabolic toxins, such as free radicals, excessive hormones and other metabolic waste).

In a healthy body, toxins get eliminated by the body systems timely and efficiently. If the body resources are depleted due to stress, illness or fatigue, the removal of toxins is slowed down leading to their accumulation in fat and bone tissues, the brain, as well as other organs and muscles. Over time it can lead to serious health problems. Clays have a wonderful ability to work with the body, gently helping to remove heavy metals and other toxic waste.

Clays, muds and salts are also wonderful natural cosmetic substances. They work on the skin by purifying it, regenerating the skin cells and improving blood circulation which ensures more nutrients reaching the skin. Oxygen gets delivered to skin cells more speedily and the removal of toxins and CO_2 is facilitated. All this brings wonderful results – the skin becomes smooth, soft, pink, glowing, wrinkles get much less visible - skin regeneration takes place.

Clays have been used by humans and animals since prehistoric times – to treat minor ailments, food poisoning, aches and pains, skin infections, mineral deficiency, in beauty rituals, as well as to make cosmetic products.

The purpose of this book is to shed light on the scientific aspects of clays and clay-like minerals and their health-enhancing properties. I hope that you find it both educational and useful in more ways than one.

Galina St George
Natural Health Practitioner
Founder of
Pure Nature Cures School of Mineral & Spa Therapies

3. Foreword

"In the sweat of thy face shalt thou eat bread, till thou return unto the ground; for out of it wast thou taken: for dust thou art, and unto dust shalt thou return". *Bible, The Book of Genesis*

Minerals are the source of life on Earth. We need them to live. Every fluid and solid matter in our body contains minerals. Every single cell needs minerals to live and reproduce. Minerals take the primary position to any nutrient available to us, since all nutrients, including vitamins, proteins, carbohydrates and fats need minerals for formation and survival. Life on Earth simply would not exist without them.

Clays are a natural source of all the minerals contained in a living organism. They have been used by all living creatures to cope with various health problems since prehistoric times. Animals eat and roll in them instinctively when they are sick, or even when healthy –to remain healthy.

Geophagy – the practice of eating clay (or 'dirt' as some call it simply) - is experiencing an unprecedented revival these days, thanks to its amazing benefits. During the First and Second World wars, many soldiers' lives have been saved by using clays internally and externally.

Health spas use muds and clays in baths, body wraps, body scrubs, masks, compresses, poultices, for the restoration of health and vitality, as well as in beauty treatments – for skin rejuvenation, detox, weight loss, and as natural ingredients to make own products. Clays differ in colour and properties, which are determined by their mineral content and chemical composition.

The earth gives us every single mineral we need. With the advancement of sophisticated medical treatments and remedies, we have lost touch with it. Opening up our minds and re-discovering the numerous powerful benefits of the simplest and most ancient remedies on Earth will help us deal with many of our problems in the most natural way.

In this book, I would like to talk about various aspects of clay science to show how and why clays are so good for us. My other goal is to look at and compare various clays and list their therapeutic benefits and applications. Having worked with clays and clay-like minerals for some time, I discovered that there is not much information which goes into detail about how they work and why they have such a powerful action on the body systems.

4. The Science of Clay

4.1. Minerals & Mineralogy

"A mineral is a naturally occurring substance formed through geological processes that has a characteristic chemical composition, a highly ordered atomic structure and specific physical properties. Klein, Cornelis and Cornelius Hurlbut, Jr. (1985) *Manual of Mineralogy*, Wiley, 20th ed.

To be classified as a mineral, a substance must be solid, formed as a result of geological processes, and have a strict crystalline structure.

Traditionally, minerals excluded any organic substances. Nowadays, many scientists agree that minerals and organic matter often come together as a result of geological processes. This has led to the following definition of minerals to be adopted by the International Mineralogical Association: "A mineral is an element or chemical compound that is normally crystalline and that has been formed as a result of geological processes."
(Source: minsocam.org/msa/ima/ima98(04).pdf Ernest H. Nickel, 1995, *The definition of a mineral*, The Canadian Mineralogist, vol. 33, pp. 689 - 690

Chemical composition and crystal structure determine the type of mineral. The crystal structure is a strict 3-dimensional arrangement of atoms which repeats itself in the same mineral. Crystal structure, like its chemical composition, determines properties of a mineral.

The graphite and diamond have the same chemical composition but different crystal structures, with carbon atoms in graphite arranged into sheets which can slide freely past each other, hence the softness of graphite. The carbon atoms in the diamond form a strong, interlocking three-dimensional network which makes it the strongest mineral in nature.

The International Mineralogical Association lists over 4,000 minerals which can contain just one, or a group of minerals. The latter is referred to as rocks or ores. Chemical composition of rocks determines what minerals would be formed as a result.

Some minerals are very stable and are not affected by the environment (e.g. granite), some, the softer and more porous varieties, are constantly changing as a result of the environmental conditions and Earth activity. Exposed to moisture, carbonic acid and other natural factors at ordinary temperatures of the Earth's surface, some of these minerals decompose and are replaced by new combinations. For example, feldspar turns into kaolinite, muscovite and quartz. These changes are accompanied by disintegration – the mineral passes into a different state – sand or earth-type which in turn may form another mineral under certain conditions. Clays are weathered sedimentary rocks. One clay type, in turn, can change into another as a result of environmental changes.

All minerals are classified according to their physical and chemical characteristics. Physical properties include their crystal structure, colour, hardness, lustre, cleavage and specific gravity. Sometimes all these properties can be determined by simply looking at the mineral. Sometimes a laboratory analysis is needed.

Minerals are subdivided into groups according to their chemical structure, or an active anion group. The largest is the silicate group which contains mainly silicium, oxygen, aluminium, magnesium, iron and calcium. Most rocks, clays and zeolite are silicates, or to be more precise - aluminosilicates. The other groups are carbonate, sulphate, halide, oxide, sulphide, phosphate, element and organic.

4.2. Clay - General Information

Clays are soft mineral substances of sedimentary or residual origin - a product of weathered volcanic ash. Various silicate minerals (quartz, micas and feldspars) which formed as a result of volcanic activity were subjected to environmental influences, both physical and chemical, and changed into clays over a long time. Clays consist of minute particles which can absorb large amounts of water. As a result, clays can be hydrated, and some clays expand on hydration. We will talk about expanding clays in more detail later.

Clays are hydrous aluminium phyllosilicates formed from other silicate minerals, such as feldspars and micas, as a result of physical and chemical alteration and weathering over billions of years.

Chemical and physical weathering of clays includes hydrolysis, leaching, oxidation, dehydration, temperature factors (heat, frost), animal activity, etc. Chemical weathering occurs under the influence of weak carbonic acid and other diluted solvents which migrate through the weathering rock.

Clays are the main constituents of sedimentary rocks – mudrocks, shales and claystones. They can also be of residual deposition and are also main constituents of soils. Some clays are formed as a result of hydrothermal activity. Clay deposits are often associated with a large lake and marine environments.

There are various clay groups, depending on their origin, chemical composition and properties. The main ones are kaolinite, smectite, illite and chlorite. Kaolinite is a white mineral formed as a result of an alteration of aluminium silicates, especially feldspars. Illite has the same constituents as kaolinite, as well as potassium. It is the main mineral of clay sediments, mudstones and shales. Illite is a type of clay formed as a result of weathering of feldspars and other silicates.

Montmorillonite (smectite group) has the same constituents as kaolinite, plus sodium and magnesium. It is derived from alteration and weathering of mafic igneous rocks. Montmorillonite is the main constituent of Fuller's earth and other smectite clays.

Certain characteristics of clays make them play a very important part in health maintenance:

1. Clays consist of minute particles below 2 μm in size, which means that their surface area is enormous and is made many times larger in certain clays on hydration. Their large surface area means that the sorption and ion exchange area in clays is very large, which is a very important property for detoxification and mineral exchange.

2. Clays have a well-researched ability to **exchange their ions** for ions of the surrounding medium.

3. **Expansion** – some clays can **expand on hydration**. This increases the surface area many times, which makes them attract even more toxic substances. Clays which expand on hydration are mainly smectites. One of the most well-known expanding minerals is montmorillonite, and some clay types have a high content of it.

4. Clays can **adsorb and absorb** the mineral and organic substances. This property is explained by the electric charge created between the clay layers, as well as on the edges of its particles. This makes clays adsorb and absorb heavy and radioactive metals, free radicals and other unwanted products of metabolic activity.

5. **Selectivity** – clays are selective as to what size ions they adsorb. Large multivalent ions (e.g. Cs) are preferred to smaller uni- (1) or bi (2)-valent ions (e.g. Li). This property is used in neutralising heavy and radioactive ions.

6. Clays act as **catalysts in organic reactions.** This property is used in reducing environmental pollution and body toxicity.

7. **The antibacterial** property of clays - clay particles are so minute that they can envelop bacteria depriving them of nutrition and oxygen, thus neutralising them (this is one of the theories for the clay's ability to neutralise germs).

People and animals have been using clays to rid themselves of infectious diseases for thousands of years. However, it has only recently been scientifically researched and publicised. This property makes clays one of the best natural antibacterial agents known to man.

"In experiments, the clay killed up to 99 per cent of superbug colonies within 24 hours. Control samples of

MRSA (methicillin-resistant Staphylococcus aureus) grew 45-fold in the same period.

The clay has a similar effect on other deadly bacteria tested, including salmonella, E. coli, and a flesh-eating disease called Buruli, a relative of leprosy which disfigures children across central and western Africa. It has been classed as "an emerging public health threat" by the World Health Organization (WHO)." (Souce: independent.co.uk/life-style/health-and-families/health-news/french-muck-is-this-the-new-penicillin-5328853.html)

8. Clays can form a **protective layer on the damaged mucous lining** which makes them important in the treatment of gastrointestinal and other disorders where mucous lining needs protection.

9. **Anti-parasite property**: clays have been used as an anti-parasite remedy for thousands of years. Exactly why and how they work in this way is not known, but both people and animals seem to benefit greatly. One theory is that they work by enveloping parasites depriving them of water and nutrition.

4.3. The Origin of Life on Earth - the "Clay Theory"

There are a lot of theories on how life on Earth started. Clay theory is one of the most exciting and interesting because of the role of minerals in the creation of life on our planet. It was developed by Dr A. Graham Cairns-Smith, an organic chemist and molecular biologist at the University of Glasgow, in 1985.

The theory is based on abiogenesis – the creation of life from non-life. The theory claims that clay can be formed from dissolved silicates. The clay crystals preserve their form during growth. The crystal shapes can change due to various external factors – physical and chemical and are replicated by other crystals of the following generations.

The crystals with the most stable growth patterns would play the dominant role in this self-replication process, and the ones with a less stable growth pattern would be suppressed by the first type. This would create a stable environment for biological life.

The second stage of this process would be the interaction of the clay environment with organic molecules – the ones that enhance the replication potential of clay crystals. The uniform shape of the crystals would be a good environment for the creation of organic molecules, and clay would act as a catalyst in this process. This would create a large number of organic molecules essential for the creation of life.

The third stage is the 'Genetic Takeover process', during which the organic molecules which used clay as a medium for growth would take over the process of self-replication from the clay crystals they used for growth, acquiring an ability to self-replicate independently.

The "clay theory" was not widely supported by the scientific circles, although it had its fans. More recently, a group of US scientists has conducted several experiments to prove this theory.

A much more recent study by a team at the Howard Hughes Medical Institute and Massachusetts General Hospital in Boston made claims that life on Earth started in the presence of clay crystals. They say that montmorillonite (of the smectite group) "not only helps form little bags of fat and liquid but helps cells use genetic material called RNA. That, in turn, is one of the key processes of life."

"They found the clay sped along the process by which fatty acids formed little bag-like structures called vesicles. The clay also carried RNA into those vesicles. A cell is, in essence, a complex bag of liquid compounds."

"Thus, we have demonstrated that not only can clay and other mineral surfaces accelerate vesicle assembly, but assuming that the clay ends up inside at least some of the time, this provides a pathway by which RNA could get into vesicles," Szostak said in a statement Thursday.

"The formation, growth and division of the earliest cells may have occurred in response to similar interactions with mineral particles and inputs of material and energy," the researchers wrote in their report, published in the journal Science. "We are not claiming that this is how life started," Szostak stressed. "We are saying that we have demonstrated growth and division without any biochemical machinery. Ultimately, if we can demonstrate more natural ways this might have happened, it may begin to give us clues about how life could have gotten started on the primitive Earth." (Source: edition.cnn.com/2003/TECH/science/10/25/clay.life.reut/index.ht ml)

Whether one chooses to believe in the clay theory or not, clay has played a crucial role in the creation and evolution of life.

4.4. History of Clay Use in Health & Beauty

Clays have been used by all living creatures since the beginning of life on Earth. Animals and birds eat clays when they are sick, roll in them to clean up their bodies, as well as to free themselves of parasites, heal wounds and ulcers.

Ancient Egyptians have been using clays for mummification. Cleopatra used clay from the Nile River and the Arabian desert in her beauty treatments. There is plentiful evidence of clay being used by ancient spas built 3000-4000 years ago. Many of these spas still exist and continue using clay.

Ancient physicians (Dioscortes, Avicenna, Galen) used clay to treat their patients for many health problems. And they did have very advanced treatments and remedies available to them.

". . . a hill in the island of Lemnos . . . in the northern Aegean Sea has produced this `earth` . . . reddish-yellow clay . . . from before Theophrastus' time (372-287 B.C.) down to the present day. According to Dana (System of Mineralogy 689), it is cimolite, a hydrous silicate of aluminium. The Ancients distinguished two kinds - one sort used as a pigment, and the other for medicinal purposes. This latter was dug with great ceremony at a certain time of the year, moulded into cubes, and stamped with a goat - the symbol of Diana. It thus became known as terra sigillata, and was an article of apothecary commerce down to the last century. It is described by Galen (xii., 12), Dioscorides (v., 63), and Pliny (xxxv., 14), as a remedy for ulcers and snake bites."

The troops of Alexander the Great and Roman soldiers used to take clays with them on long marches to ward off hunger and food poisoning.

American Indians used and are still using clays in spiritual ceremonies and healing procedures. African tribes used and are still using clay for similar purposes. African women have been observed to eat "dirt" when pregnant or lactating. In societies which have not lost touch with nature, clay takes a very high position as a healing, preventative remedy and food. Clay is also used for water purification where clean water is difficult or impossible to obtain.

For generations, clay has been eaten by starving nations at times of hunger. Even now in poorer countries clays (mud pies) are made and eaten when food is short (Philippines, New Guinea,

Costa Rica, Guatemala and the Amazon and Orinoco basins of South America).

I have recently come across an article about pregnant women in Haiti eating mud pies. There are arguments that the mud pies are a tradition in certain nations and are eaten as a natural mineral supplement.

Throughout the two World wars clays were part of Russian, French and German soldiers' rations to prevent and treat food poisoning, diarrhoea, as well as wound infections. Many lives and limbs have been saved by humble clay.

"Under the name of 'Cutler's earth' clay was used in some districts of France – and perhaps it is still used – as a resolutive and against burns from first to the third degree. It is also known under the names of Luvos, aluminium silicate, colloidal white clay, balus, and others." (Our Earth, Our Cure by Raymond Dextreit, 1993, p.14).

German naturopaths Kneipp, Kuhn, Felke and Just used clays for medicinal purposes. Father Kneipp used clay and vinegar poultices in his practice – a remedy still used in naturopathic practices today. Another German naturopath Professor Julius

Stumpf treated Asiatic cholera when antibiotics such as penicillin had to wait for a few more decades to appear.

Bentonite clay and zeolite were used in Ukraine to decontaminate the area after the Chernobyl nuclear disaster. Huge amounts were used to bury the reactors. They were also given to the firefighters and the local population in the form of galettes to take radioactive elements and heavy metals out of the body.

In Russia clays, alongside muds, have been used at medical spas, resorts and sanatoria to treat chronic and acute diseases for centuries. European, Mediterranean resorts are famous for using clays too. Clays, especially the ones extracted from salt lakes, are used to treat psoriasis, eczema, musculoskeletal, genitourinary, circulation and numerous other disorders.

Clays are routinely used and prescribed both by doctors and naturopaths for many health conditions in France. French clays are very well known and valued among clay users, as well as drugs and cosmetics manufacturers. Recently, French Green clay has been popularised by the Independent newspaper in the UK as an effective antibiotic against hospital superbugs.
(Source: independent.co.uk/life-style/health-and-families/health-news/french-muck-is-this-the-new-penicillin-5328853.html)

The late French doctor, Lyne Brunet de Courssu, successfully treated many of her patients in Ivory Coast (Africa) for a horrific flesh-eating disease - Buruli ulcers – with French Green Clays. The results were staggering even in the most advanced cases. The work is now being continued by her son and colleagues.

4.5. More about Geophagy

People and animals have been eating clay since prehistoric times. The attraction to clay is instinctive. Our ancestors, without much thinking, ate clay to stop themselves being poisoned, to treat diarrhoea, wounds, aches and pains, facilitate birth, supplement themselves with minerals, suppress hunger and what not. They also attributed magic properties to clay and used it in all sorts of spiritual ceremonies. This tradition is still very much alive in tribal environments where clay is treated as a sacred remedy.

"Examination of the diets of certain tribes in the high Andes of South America and Central Africa, and those of Australian aborigines, showed that these people use clay to avoid getting stomach-ache, dysentery, and food infections. Indeed, the Quetchus Indians of South America used to dip their potatoes into an aqueous suspension of clay, immediately before eating, to prevent the build-up of acidity in the stomach.

This dietetic procedure is still being followed by some tribes of American Indians. A similar practice was traditionally carried out onboard ships where sailors used clays not only to adsorb odours and moisture but also to treat dysentery, burns, boils, sore mouths, and other internal and external disorders." (Source: Clays and Clay Minerals as Drugs, M.T. Droy-Lefaix and F.Tateo, Beaufour-IPSEN, F-75016 Paris, France; Instituto do Ricerca sulle Argillle, CNR, I-85050 Tito Scalo (PZ), Italy – Handbook of Clay Science, p. 743, ISBN 0080441831, F.Bergaya, B.K.G.Theng and G.Lagaly).

Jared Diamond in his article "Eat Dirt" (Discover magazine, 1988) investigated reasons for geophagy in animals and humans which he observed on his trips. "Why should anyone-person, ungulate, or bird-eat soil? And how do dirt eaters choose which soil to consume? Why do plant-eating animals and pregnant or nursing women particularly hunger for soil?

You might suppose the easiest way to get answers would be to ask people since animals can't tell us. But if you quiz soil-eating people about their motives, they just give unhelpful replies like "I feel good when I eat it" or "I like the taste." If you press them, they say they think it cures stomach problems or worms or diarrhoea or aids, or that it is good for them during pregnancy, or that it adds a good taste to food or masks bitter tastes, or that it is useful as a pacifier in a baby's mouth.

These varied answers don't identify precise physiological explanations for geophagy, but they suggest several possible benefits. The six explanations most discussed among zoologists, anthropologists, and doctors are to assuage hunger, to provide grit for grinding food in the stomach, to buffer stomach contents, to cure diarrhoea, to serve as a mineral supplement, and to adsorb toxins".

He then talks about each theory in more detail and seems to be inclined to accept the detoxification theory for geophagy as the dominant one, based on his observations of the American Indians who added clay to various toxic foods aiming to neutralize.

It seems to me that for most people using clay, attraction to this humble mineral bypasses consciousness and exists on a very deep, primitive level which does not have much to do with the rational thinking. People who eat clay cannot explain why they are doing it. They just know it is good for them and source the best clay they can find, especially if clay consumption has been a tradition passed from one generation to another.

Because of this instinctive craving, those of us who use rationality as the main guide for choosing our remedies often get perplexed by the idea of eating something which is not a food. I see distrustful faces sometimes when I mention that I drink clay.

With scientific progress, we have forgotten many things which have been in everyday use for thousands of years. Developments in the allopathic medicine have played a huge role in us losing touch with natural remedies our ancestors have been using. The 20th century brought us penicillin and many other medicines which have saved a lot of lives. Scientists have developed medicines for any illness.

In the meantime, the knowledge of the wonders of traditional, non-medical remedies like clay has been lost. Forgotten is the fact that doctors as recently as in the first 5 decades of the 20th century were using clays to save lives – during both world wars. Clay was considered so important that soldiers – Russian, German & French – were issued clay rations for internal and external use. Soldiers were eating clay to stop diarrhoea, infections, prevent food poisoning and to satisfy hunger.

Clays are routinely eaten by people in Asia, Africa and South America nowadays. Mud pies are made out of clay, salt and water, baked and eaten by people not just when there is not enough food going round, but because it is part of these people's diet and lifestyle. One can guess that they are only healthier for it, since not only clay provides important minerals, but it also rids the organism of all kinds of infections, poisons and keeps parasites at bay.

In the west, clays are commonly used in France. Smectite clays can be found at pharmacies, and doctors prescribe them for stomach problems and infections. Clays are being sold at health shops in the UK and the US as well.

Kaolinite, the white clay, has been used in medications for stomach problems, diarrhoea and other remedies for generations. It is classified as a sorbent in the pharmaceutical industry. Fullers Earth of the smectite group is used in the food and wine industry. It is also good clay for eating since it is very close in composition to calcium bentonite. Other clays which are popular for eating are calcium bentonite, sodium bentonite, French green montmorillonite and French green illite. There are also varieties of these clays which are offered by various manufacturers worldwide.

So clays are already eaten by us - whether we are aware of it or not. We just need to eat them consciously, since the impact from using clays on a conscious level is not purely physical, but also psychological and spiritual, reconnecting us with nature and our wild roots which go millions of years back.

If you decide to try, I suggest that you choose a supplier who can provide you with the datasheets for their product. You need to pay particular attention to the content of heavy metals and bacteriological data.

For your information, ALL clays contain heavy metals and some contain a certain amount of live matter (bacteria, fungi, spores). Clays don't normally release heavy metals into the body, due to the strength of ionic bonds within the clay structure. These bonds require strong chemicals (e.g. acids) to be broken. However, it is best to look for a product where heavy metal content is within reasonable limits.

You can find information about permitted limits for food products in your country from your local food standards agency. However, one should keep in mind that clays are naturally mined substances and that it would not always be possible to achieve consistency in the chemical data even within the same batch, let alone the same supply.

4.6. Structure and Catalytic Properties of Clay

A typical clay particle is normally very small - <2μm, which results in the presence of very large surface areas. Clay minerals are composed of silicium, aluminium or magnesium ion or both, and water. Iron can be a substitute for aluminium and magnesium, and potassium, sodium, and calcium are often present in abundant quantities as well.

Clays consist of continuous two-dimensional sheets of corner-sharing SiO_4 and AlO_4 tetrahedra which share three apical (corner-positioned) oxygen atoms, with the fourth remaining unshared and pointing in the same direction. As a result, they form hexagonal sheets which in clays are bonded to octahedral sheets composed of aluminium or magnesium cations. This bonding leads to distortions in clay structure which leads to changes in the properties of clays.

Depending on how sheets of corner-sharing SiO4 and AlO4 tetrahedra are packaged into layers, clays can have a 1:1 and 2:1 structure. Kaolinite clays have a 1:1 structure with one tetrahedral silica sheet and one octahedral alumina sheet, and smectites have a 2:1 structure, where two tetrahedral silica sheets with the unshared vertex (corner oxygen) of each sheet pointing towards each other and forming each side of the octahedral alumina sheet.

The ions (anions) at the exposed surface of the octahedral sheet are hydroxyls. The 1:1 structure of kaolinite clays does not allow for expansion. The oxygen ions of the tetrahedral sheet bind to the hydroxyl ions of the octahedral sheet of the consecutive layer. Unlike smectites, there is no electrical charge and no molecules or cations between the layers in the kaolinite group.

 In the 2:1 structure, the silicate layer consists of one octahedral alumina sheet sandwiched by two tetrahedral silica sheets that are oriented in opposite directions.

Both illite and smectite clays have a 2:1 structure. Illite is of sedimentary origin and belongs to the mica group. It is characterised by numerous structural irregularities, with numerous stacking disorders – the layers are virtually piled on top of each other in quite a chaotic manner. Unlike the smectite clays, illite does not swell on hydration.

"The distinguishing feature of the smectite structure is that water and other polar molecules (in the form of certain organic substances) can, by entering between the unit layers, cause the structure to expand... Thus this dimension may vary from about 9.6 Å, when there are no polar molecules between the unit layers, to nearly complete separation of the individual layers" of the clay mineral. (2008). Encyclopaedia Britannica. Retrieved August 07, 2008, from Encyclopaedia Britannica Online: (Souce: britannica.com/EBchecked/topic/120723/clay-mineral)

One of the most interesting and effective clay minerals which are present both in bentonite and Fuller's Earth is montmorillonite. It has a high expansion and ion exchange capacity and is very active as a catalyst in organic reactions – the property which is widely used to control environmental pollution and toxicity.

Structurally, montmorillonite is composed of a sheet of octahedrally coordinated gibbsite [$Al2(OH)6$] positioned between two sheets of tetrahedrally coordinated silicate [$SiO4$]4-sheets. The interlayer sheet determines the physical and chemical properties of the mineral.

The most important property of montmorillonite is its high cation exchange capacity which happens because of Al^{3+} exchanges for Si^{4+} in the tetrahedral sheets, and of Mg^{2+} cations exchange for Al^{3+} cations in the octahedral sheets, thus creating a charge imbalance. The defects at the edges of clay layers add to this imbalance. The balancing cations of Na^+, Ca^{2+} and Mg^{2+} are situated between the clay layers. The layers move apart on hydration which leads to the clay swelling and the existing interlayer cations becoming easily exchangeable.

Na^+, Ca^{2+} and Mg^{2+} act as compensatory cations for the charge imbalance. When the clay is dry, the balancing interlayer cations of Na^+, Ca^{2+} and Mg^{2+} reside in the hexagonal cavities of the silica sheets. However, when it is hydrated, the cations position themselves between the lamellae (thin plate-like structures) and become exchangeable by a variety of cations – metallic and non-metallic, organic and inorganic, such as H_3O^+, NH_4^+, Al^{3+}, Fe^{3+} and others.

This property of montmorillonite is very important in reducing the environmental pollution. To enhance its catalytic property, clays are treated, or activated, to become more acidic and therefore more active.

For health purposes, activated clays cannot be used. However, activation is not needed for clay to do its wonderful job in reducing the body 'pollution', or toxicity – its natural catalytic properties are more than sufficient for this purpose.

4.7. Ion (Cation) Exchange

To understand why and how clays work and why they are so good for us, it is very important to understand what happens on a very basic, molecular level when they are in contact with liquids.

Our bodies contain 45-75% of water, depending on the amount of body fat, and both ion exchange and sorption are integral functions which are part of the body metabolism and without which we could not exist. Ion exchange plays a crucial part in body detoxification. It is used in many industries. Some of them are water purification, agricultural soil enrichment, odour control, site decontamination from radioactive waste, etc.

Clays possess a property called 'ion exchange'. It is also referred to as 'cation', 'anion', 'ionic' and 'cationic' exchange, depending on the charge of the ions exchanged (positive or negative). Ion is a general term for charged minute particles which form a molecule. They can be either cations or anions.

Cations are positively charged ions, and anions are negatively charged ones. Ions can only exist in a liquid environment since they need water to break away from a molecule and react with other ions. Ion exchange is a very important property - it makes clays active.

Ion exchange is a process during which ions from a liquid solution exchange with ions of a solid substance of mineral (e.g. clays) or organic (e.g. resins) origin. Removed ions are replaced by equivalent amounts of other ions of the same charge.

Depending on the charge of the exchanged and exchanging ions, the process can be called the cationic or anionic exchange. During cationic exchange positively charged ions – cations – of a solution replace positively charged ions of the solid substance, due to a greater affinity of the substance with the cations of the solution. Anionic exchange is the same process for negatively charged ions.

Each mineral has a certain capacity for ion exchange. Encyclopaedia Britannica defines it as a "measure of the ability of an insoluble material to undergo displacement of ions previously attached and loosely incorporated into its structure by oppositely charged ions present in the surrounding solution... High cation-exchange capacities are characteristic of clay minerals and numerous other natural and synthetic substances possessing ion-exchanging properties". **Ion-exchange capacity**. (2008). In Encyclopedia *Britannica*. Retrieved July 04, 2008, from Encyclopaedia Britannica Online (Source: britannica.com/EBchecked/topic/292789/ion-exchange-capacity)

Cation Exchange Capacity (CEC) is usually expressed in milliequivalents (meq) /100g. CEC of clays and clay minerals is defined as the number of cations available for exchange at a certain pH – normally 7 (neutral). Cation exchange capacity depends on several factors: the size of the particles (smaller particles will have a higher CEC than larger ones), temperature, the concentration of the solution etc. Clays display a strong preference for organic cations over inorganic ones, which also plays a very important role in body detoxification from organic toxins.

The range of the cation-exchange capacities of the clay minerals is given in the Table – "Cation-exchange capacities and specific surface areas of clay minerals".

Mineral	Cation exchange capacity at pH 7 (milliequivalents per 100 grams)	Specific surface area (square meters per gram)
Kaolinite	3–15	5–40
Halloysite (hydrated)	40–50	1,100*
Illite	10–40	10–100
Chlorite	10–40	10–55
Vermiculite	100–150	760*
Smectite	80–120	40–800
Palygorskite-sepiolite	3–20	40–180
Allophane	30–135	2,200*
Imogolite	20–30	1,540*
*Upper limit of estimated values.		

Clay Mineral. (2008). In Encyclopedia *Britannica*. Retrieved July 04, 2008, from Encyclopedia Britannica Online. (Source: britannica.com/EBchecked/topic/120723/clay-mineral)

Here is what Dorothy Carroll says about ion exchange in her article "Ion exchange in clays and other minerals":

"Ion exchange in clays and other minerals is dependent on the crystalline structure of the mineral and the chemical composition of any solution in contact with the mineral... Ion exchange in these minerals is a reversible chemical reaction that takes place between ions held near a mineral surface by unbalanced electrical charges within the mineral framework and ions in a solution in contact with the mineral. Generally, the excess charge on the mineral is negative, and it attracts cations from the solution to neutralize this charge.

Chemical reactions in the ion exchange follow the law of mass action, but the reactions are restricted by the number of exchange sites on the mineral and by the strength of the bonding of the exchangeable cations to the mineral surface. Titration of H-clays with bases shows that montmorillonite and illite clays behave like a mixture of 2 or 3 different acids, whereas kaolinite, with an indefinite number of exchange sites, behaves like an indefinite number of acids.

Ion-exchange capacity is measured in chemical equivalents of base adsorbed at pH 7. Each clay mineral has a range of exchange capacities because of differences in structure and chemical composition. The ranges (in milliequivalents per 100 grams) are kaolinite, 3-15; halloysite ($2H_2O$), 5-10; halloysite ($4H_2O$), 40-50; montmorillonite, 70-100; "illite", 10-40; vermiculite, 100-150; glauconite, 11-20; attapulgite, 20-30; and allophane, 70. The common metallic cations found in exchange positions in clay minerals are Ca (super +2) , Mg (super +2) , Na (super +) , and K (super +) . At low pH values H (super +) replaces other cations. The order of replaceability of the common cations has been found to be: Li (super +) < Na (super +) < K (super +) < Rb (super +) < Cs (super +) and Mg (super +2) < Ca (super +2) < Sr (super +2) < Ba (super +2) . Bivalent cations enter the exchange sites preferentially to univalent cations. The common exchangeable cation in most clay minerals in soils is Ca (super +2) . " (Source: bulletin.geoscienceworld.org/cgi/content/abstract/70/6/749).

4.8. Adsorption, Absorption & Intercalation

Ion exchange is closely linked to the processes of **sorption** and **intercalation**. There are 2 basic types of sorption – **ad**sorption and **ab**sorption. There is also **de**sorption – a process which reverses the other two.

Adsorption describes the attachment of substances to the surface of a mineral due to their opposite electric charge. In clays, this process involves neutral species (H2O, H4SiO4), organic molecules and ions.

"Depending on deficiency in the positive or negative charge balance (locally or overall) of mineral structures, clay minerals can adsorb certain cations and anions and retain them around the outside of the structural unit in an exchangeable state, generally without affecting the basic silicate structure. These adsorbed ions are easily exchanged by other ions. The exchange reaction differs from simple sorption because it has a quantitative relationship between reacting ions.

Absorption is a deeper process of 'ingestion' of an ion or organic molecule by a molecular structure of a mineral (e.g. into zeolite channels, or spaces between clay sheets). All these processes are possible because of ion activity between minerals and the surrounding environment.

Intercalation is a variety of adsorption where organic molecules penetrate between the layers of clay. It is an important process in detoxification. Kaolin, for example, can adsorb "particular types of neutral organic compounds between the layers... Intercalated guest molecules can be displaced by other suitable molecules... The interlayer cations can be exchanged by various types of organic cations. " (Clay Mineral Organic Interactions, G.Lagaly, M.Ogawa and I.Dekany - The Book of Clay Science, V.1, p. 309, F.Bergaya, B.K.G.Theng, G.Lagaly, 2008).

Like sorption, intercalation is a reversible process – organic substances can be washed out by water or replaced by other ions. Intercalation is a process typical of most clays, including kaolinites and smectites, although the degree of intercalation is not the same for clays taken from different sources and depends on many factors which are mainly determined by the composition of the clay mineral. Intercalation can take place between clays on the one side and polar (charged) and neutral molecules on the other. Both dry and hydrated clays can intercalate guest substances.

Also, organic compounds can be intercalated into clays from dry, liquid and solid states. Where a neutral molecule is intercalated, it is placed between the layers as a result of the stepwise expansion of the layers of clay (as in expanding smectites). Intercalated molecules/ions can be displaced by other ions if they form a closer affinity with the clay.

4.9. Hydration & Expansion of Clays

Sorption is closely linked to clay hydration. The way clays are hydrated depends on their structure and the strength of interlayer ionic bonds. With the weaker bond, like in smectite clays, hydration is much higher than in illite and kaolinite clay types.

Even within the same clay group, there are distinctions, depending on the source of clay and its composition. Montmorillonite clay, for example, has very high hydration capacity, and so does sodium bentonite.

Hydration, in turn, leads to expansion of a clay mineral and a dramatic increase of the surface which can interact with the environment in terms of ionic exchange and sorption of inorganic and organic toxins.

"In a theoretical study of water molecules clustered near the siloxane surface of kaolinite, the water molecules had a tendency to avoid this surface consistent with its hydrophobic character (Nulens et al, 1998).

In contrast, the presence of hydrated cations, such as Na^+, K^+, Mg^{2+} and Ca^{2+}, in the interlayer region of smectites and vermiculites impart an overall hydrophilic nature to these clay minerals. The hydration dynamics of these cations and the interaction of water with these metal ions underlie many important processes associated with clay minerals including their ability to swell in water.

Expandable clay minerals are known to be strongly hydrophilic and this is largely attributed to the hydration of certain inorganic cations (Sposito and Prost, 1982; Jouany and Chassin, 1987; Johnson et al, 1992, Xu et al, 2000). Also, the hydroxylated surface of gibbsite and the gibbsite-like surface of kaolinite have some hydrophilic character (Source: Nulen et al, 1998, Surface and Interface Chemistry of Clay Minerals, R.A.Schoonheidt and C.T.Johnston – Handbook of Clay Science, F. Bergaya, B.K.G.Theng and G.Lagaly, 2008, p.96).

Smectites can absorb up to half of their mass in water, and their interaction with water depends on the nature of exchangeable cations.

In smectites and vermiculites, hydration happens as a result of the attraction of water molecules to exchangeable cations in clays (hydrophilic property). The water absorbed between the layers of smectite is different from the bulk water since water molecules between clay layers are polarised both by the interlayer cations and are bound to a negative centre by a hydrogen bridge. As a result, the interlayer water becomes more acidic. This leads to water molecules being trapped between the layers, and as a result, the clay expands on hydration.

With kaolinite, there is some attraction of water molecules to the surface ions, but overall the clay is largely hydrophobic, which means that the clay does not expand.

4.10. The selectivity of Clays & Heavy Metals

Clay minerals are selective as to what size ions they will absorb – a very important factor in detoxification and understanding why clays play such an important role in natural health care. Larger ions are preferred in this case to smaller ones. The binding selectivity of clays is expressed in the Handbook of Clay Science as a binding coefficient. Here are some of the data:

$Li+$ - 0.6, $Na+$ - 1, $K+$ - 2, $Cs+$ - 200, Mg^{2+} - 2, Ca^{2+} - 4-40, Sr^{2+} - 5, Cd^{2+} - 10, $MB+$ - 108, $TFT+$ - 109.

This means that the heavy ions of cadmium (a heavy metal which gets into our bodies through smoking and pollution) are absorbed by clay in preference to the light ions of lithium and potassium.

For smectites, this preference is expressed in the following order:

$Cs+ > Rb+ > K+ > Na+ > Li+$ and
$Mg^{2+} > Ca^{2+} \approx Sr^{2+} \approx Ba^{2+}$

Caesium ions are thus preferred to Lithium ions between the layers, although the edges of the clay crystals do not show the same preference.

"The preference of clay minerals for certain cations is caused by several effects. These include hydration of the cations at the surface and in solution (entropy!), electrostatic cation-surface and cation-cation interactions between the water molecules and the surface and the polarizability or hard and soft acid-base (HSAB) character of the cations (Xu and Harsh, 1992; Auboiroux et al, 1998 -
Handbook of Clay Science, F. Bergaya, B.K.G.Theng and G.Lagaly, 2008, p.985).

This preference means that clays attract large ions of heavy metals in preference to smaller ions important for normal body functioning. The number of heavy metal cations absorbed often exceeds the cationic exchange capacity of the clay mineral.

Clays can also exchange anions, but on a much smaller scale. "For anions, such as chloride and nitrate, the anion exchange capacity amounts to a few cmo (-)/kg. By contrast, up to 20-30 cmo(-)/kg of phosphate and arsenate (cations – G.G.) can be absorbed by kaolinite and montmorillonite (Muljadi et al, 1966a, 1966b, 1966c, Grim, 1968 - Handbook of Clay Science, F. Bergaya, B.K.G.Theng and G.Lagaly, 2008, p.987).

5. Clay Groups

Clays differ in structure and composition. Just like there are no two identical fingerprints, it is impossible to find two identical clays - they come from different sources, and clay from each source has its own mineralogical composition. Also, clays are rarely found as pure minerals. Most deposits contain a number of minerals, with one group or type dominating the others. Smectite clay may have a certain percentage of kaolinite, illite, montmorillonite and micas.

"The SiO2 ratio ... is the key factor determining clay mineral types. These minerals can be classified based on variations of chemical composition and atomic structure into nine groups: (1) kaolin-serpentine (kaolinite, halloysite, lizardite, chrysotile), (2) pyrophyllite-talc, (3) mica (illite, glauconite, celadonite), (4) vermiculite, (5) smectite (montmorillonite, nontronite, saponite), (6) chlorite (sudoite, clinochlore, chamosite), (7) sepiolite-palygorskite, (8) interstratified clay minerals (*e.g.,* rectorite, corrensite, tosudite), and (9) allophane-imogolite ". (2008). Encyclopedia *Britannica*. Retrieved August 07, 2008, from Encyclopedia Britannica Online: (Source: britannica.com/science/clay-mineral)

We shall look at three main clay groups which have practical applications in medicine, health and beauty – **kaolinite** (kaolin-serpentine group), **montmorillonite** (smectite group) and **illite** (mica group). Each group includes clays of different chemical composition from different sources. It is the predominant mineral which determines the name of a clay. However, clays from any two sources will most certainly differ both in mineral and chemical composition, as well as physical properties. This is why red illite clay from one source will even visually be different from red illite clay from another source. They will also have other differences too. And even clays from the same deposit may differ, depending on the layer they have come from, and surrounding minerals.

5.1. The Kaolinite Group

Kaolinite is a layered aluminosilicate mineral with the 1:1 structure - one tetrahedral silica sheet linked to 1 octahedral alumina sheet via oxygen atoms. Its chemical formula is $Al_2Si_2O_5(OH)_4$. The most common clay which belongs to this group is kaolin or china clay. Kaolin is named after a hill in China – Kao-Ling – where it was first mined. It is now mined in Brazil, France, UK, Germany, China, Australia, USA and other countries.

It is soft, chalky and can be white, pink, yellow, orange and even red (depending on its chemical composition), of sedimentary origin, formed as a result of weathering of aluminosilicate minerals such as feldspar and hydrothermal decomposition of granite rocks. Most deposits contain only a certain proportion of kaolinite, with the remainder consisting of feldspar, mica, muscovite and quartz.

Kaolin has low hydration capacity – it does not swell in water, due to stronger attraction between the layers, since its interlayer charge is balanced, which does not allow the layers to separate. Its cation exchange capacity is also low – normally 1-15 meq/100g (but can be higher depending on its origin and mineral composition), due to a much lower quantity of active interlayer cations than in smectite clays. It is highly sorbent.

Kaolin applications in health are based around its powerful ability to adsorb harmful inorganic and organic substances – heavy metals, paraquat (commercially used herbicide – extremely poisonous to humans and animals if swallowed), oil, proteins, and also bacteria, viruses (Steel & Anderson, 1972, Lipson & Stotzky, 1983).

Unlike smectite clays, it attracts particles only to its surface (adsorption), and not between the layers, so the particles can be easily removed from kaolin's surface. Due to its adsorbent, coating and bulk-forming properties, kaolin is used in anti-diarrhoea medications (Kaopectate) and stomach-soothing remedies.

The cosmetic industry is its other big user – kaolin is used to manufacture powders, creams and lotions, soaps, mascara, toothpaste, etc. It also makes gentle, soothing, cleansing, adsorbing masks.

5.2. The Smectite Group

The smectite clays were formed as a result of sedimentation of volcanic ash in the soil, rocks, sea beds and water beds. They are the most abundant clays found in nature.

They are 2:1 minerals. The most well-known clays in the smectite group are Fuller's earth, calcium Bentonite (the closest relative of Fuller's earth, with the only difference that the main exchangeable ion in it is calcium as opposed to magnesium in Fuller's earth) and sodium bentonite. Montmorillonite is the main component in the clays of this group.

Smectite clays have very high swelling and ionic exchange capacity and therefore a wide range of applications – industrial, cosmetic, medical and medicinal, in the food industry, agriculture, etc. The high cation exchange capacity is explained by the substitution in the structural lattice of the silicon ions, with cations creating a strong negative surface charge which is balanced by interlayer cations $Na+$, $Ca2+$, $K+$, $Mg2+$. These cations are exchangeable, due to their loose binding, which explains the high ionic exchange capacity of these clays.

The most well-known clays of the smectite group are calcium bentonite, sodium bentonite, Fuller's earth, French green montmorillonite and variations of the bentonite clays from quarries all over the world. Many of these clays are used for medicinal purposes.

1. Calcium bentonite is non-swelling clay which has double water layer particles with $Ca2+$ as the main exchangeable ion. It has a high cation exchange rate and is a very popular type of clay in detoxification procedures.

2. Sodium bentonite is swelling clay which has single water layer particles containing $Na+$ (sodium) as the

exchangeable ion. It swells up to 15 times when hydrated, and this property makes it very useful in the oil drilling industry. In health, sodium bentonite can be used to great effect in detoxification, healing of ulcers, addressing excessive body acidity and associated conditions.

3. Fuller's earth is naturally bleaching, similar in structure and properties to calcium bentonite, with magnesium, sodium and calcium being exchangeable ions. Montmorillonite is the principal clay mineral in Fuller's earth. It may also contain kaolinite, attapulgite and other minerals, which explains its variable chemical composition and properties. It has a variety of applications in the health and beauty industry, due to its high ion exchange and sorptive properties.

Sodium or calcium in the bentonite clays is exchanged for magnesium or iron. All the bentonite clays and Fuller's earth have a very high cationic exchange and sorption capacity and are therefore valuable industrial clays. These properties also make them very popular in the cosmetics and beauty industries, food and wine manufacture, and increasingly as medicinal clays.

Bentonite clays are also called **montmorillonite** clays due to a high level of montmorillonite. Montmorillonite is a soft mineral with high expanding capacity when hydrated. It was first discovered in Montmorillon region in France.

Encyclopaedia Britannica defines montmorillonite the following way: "any of a group of clay minerals and their chemical varieties that swell in water and possess high cation-exchange capacities. The theoretical formula for montmorillonite (*i.e.,* without structural substitutions) is $(OH)4\ Si8\ Al4\ O20 \cdot nH2\ O$".

Montmorillonite particles are extremely small. They take up water between their layers, which leads to the swelling of the mineral on hydration. Montmorillonite also has a very high cationic exchange capacity. Its high sorptive and ionic exchange capacity is passed on to the smectite clays containing montmorillonite – bentonite clays and Fuller's earth.

These properties are widely used in numerous industries, beauty and health care. The ability of montmorillonite to exchange minerals within its structure for environmental minerals and toxic organic substances is a very valuable property used in detoxification of the environment and human/animal organism.

5.3. The Illite Group

The illite group is named after the state of Illinois where it was first identified. Illite is a non-expanding mineral. The chemical formula: $(K,H3O)(Al,Mg,Fe)2(Si,Al)4O10[(OH)2,(H2O)$. Illite is a layered silicate (phyllosilicate).

The best-known species of illite is glauconite, which is a type of green mineral clay. It is typically found in clays of marine origin. Other colours include white and yellow. Unlike the smectite clays, illite clays do not expand when hydrated. They are, however, highly sorbent, taking water into numerous pores of their crystalline structure.

Illite clays occur as aggregates of small grey to white crystals. Illite is the product of weathering of muscovite and feldspar. Structurally, illite consists of tiny irregular platelets of uncertain morphology. It is common in soils and rocks of sedimentary origin. Illite clays are rich in iron, potassium and many other macro- and micro- minerals. Alongside montmorillonite, illite clays have very potent therapeutic properties and are used to treat a wide variety of problems. They are also very popular in the manufacture of cosmetics and beauty industry.

6. Colours of the Rainbow

6.1. Blue Cambrian Clay

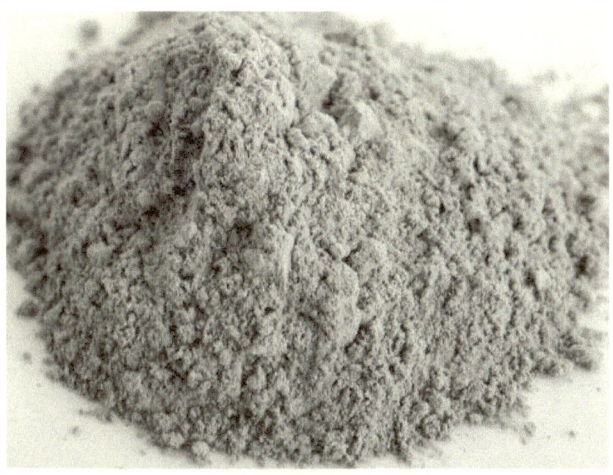

Blue clay - a member of the smectite group - is considered to be the most potent of all medicinal clays. Like with all minerals, the quality and composition of the deposit will vary greatly. Blue clay contains several minerals in their natural colloidal form which are used by the body to produce enzymes and in many other bodily functions. It is a rich source of trace minerals, with the highest ability to adsorb and absorb, so it is one of the most popular bulking agents in the beauty industry.

Being highly potent, it has some of the most powerful detoxifying properties of all clays. Blue and red montmorillonite clays have similar properties and benefits. Blue clay is very effective at drawing oils and toxins from the skin. It is also an excellent remedy for acne, arthritis, toxicity, aches and pains, mineral deficiencies, ulcers, and whatnot. Blue clay is found mainly in Russia and some parts of Eastern Europe.

6.2. Red Montmorillonite Clay

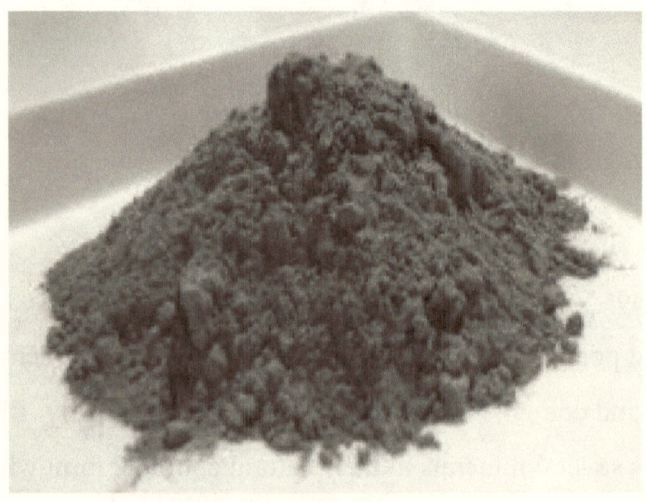

Red montmorillonite is a close relative of blue montmorillonite and is highly efficient at drawing oils and toxins from the skin. It can also be used to soothe sore muscles, sprains, bruises and more.

In the cosmetic industry, it used in soaps and body/foot powders as a natural colour additive. This is also very popular clay in natural medicine for its detoxifying qualities. It is good to use in baths, compresses, face masks and body wraps.

6.3. Bentonite Clays

Bentonite includes 2 types of clay – calcium and sodium bentonite - which both belong to the smectite group. It is also called "montmorillonite clay", due to a high content of montmorillonite in it. It is also sometimes referred to as "montmorillonite".

Bentonite clay owes its name to a place called Fort Benton in the USA. It was formed by an alteration of volcanic glass to clay minerals which are less than .005mm in size. It consists of hydrous aluminium silicates, plus iron oxide and magnesium oxide, as well as either sodium or calcium oxide. It can absorb 40 - 50 times its weight and swells to form a gel-like mass. This clay is often used for drawing poultices and for treating sprains, bruises, insect bites, rashes, in perspiration absorbing foot powders, in exfoliating and detoxifying face masks and body wraps.

6.4. Calcium Bentonite Clay

Calcium bentonite is a natural mineral clay composed mainly of aluminium, silica, iron oxides, lime, magnesium, and water in extremely variable proportions. It is generally classified as sedimentary clay. In colour, it may be whitish, buff, brown, green, olive, or blue.

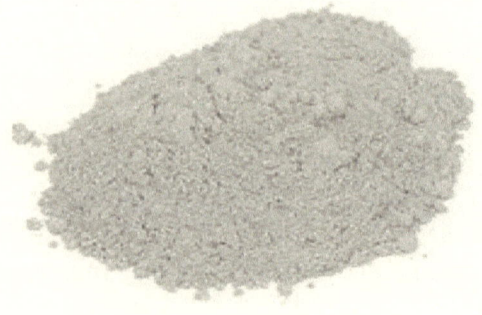

Calcium is the main exchangeable ion in this clay, hence the name. It has a high cation exchange rate and close to neutral pH.

This clay is widely used in healing and is one of the most popular clays in detox procedures.

6.5. Fuller's Earth

Fuller's earth is a close relative of calcium bentonite. Both have strong bleaching properties, due to their high ion exchange capacity. Both have montmorillonite as the main constituent. The only difference is that it has magnesium as the main exchangeable ion, while calcium bentonite has calcium as the main exchangeable ion.

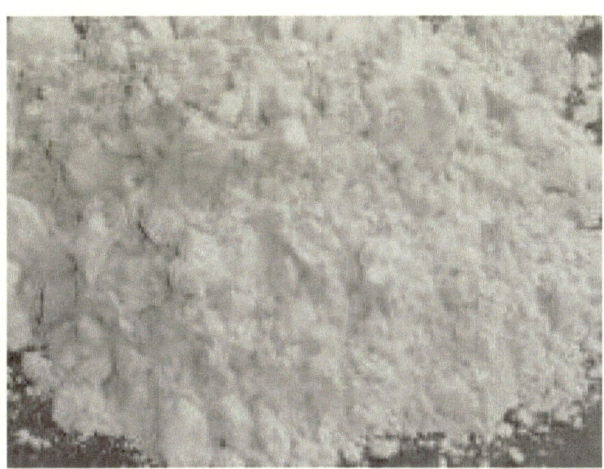

Fuller's earth was originally used in the fulling of wool to remove oil and grease but is now used in refining edible oils. It is also a useful base ingredient for facial clay recipes.

Fuller's earth is widely used in face masks for oily and blemished skin, due to its drying effect. It is highly sorbent and is great for treating conditions where drying is required. It is an excellent choice of clay for detoxification.

6.6. Sodium Bentonite Clay

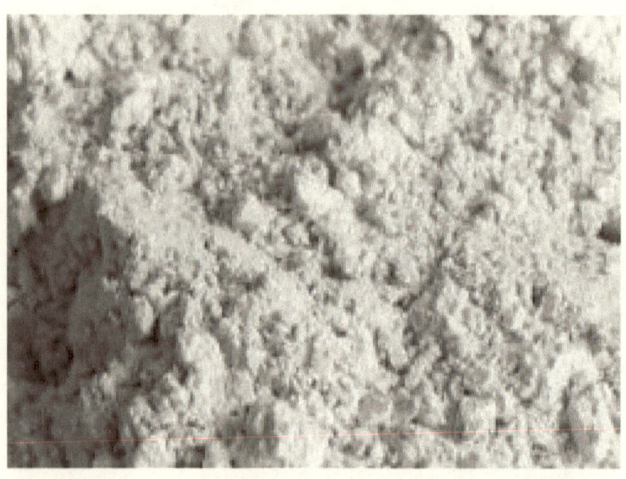

Sodium bentonite is part of the smectite group of clays. It has a 2:1 structure, expands on hydration (up to 15 times) and has very high cationic exchange capacity, with sodium being the main exchangeable ion. Sodium bentonite is highly alkaline clay, with an average pH of 9-10. It is a great clay for treating ulcers, infections and many ailments connected with high acidity. This clay is not easily mixed with water, so patience and time are needed when doing it. When hydrated, it feels like soap. Sodium bentonite has a high cation exchange rate.

6.7. Glacier Clay

Glacier clay (also known as Canadian Glacial Clay) is a rare type of clay found in British Columbia. It contains over 30 minerals and trace elements of less than .15 micron particle size making it one of the finest glacial marine clays discovered in the world. It has a natural pH balance of 6.5 to 7.3.

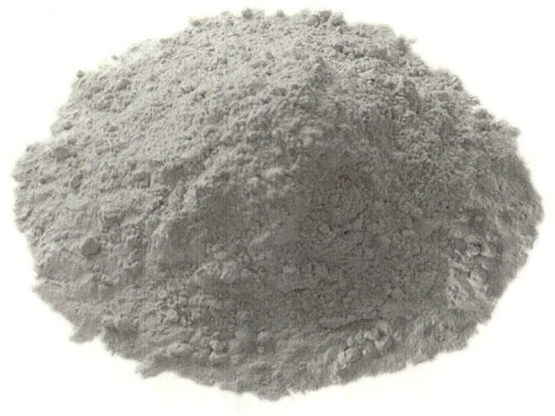

It is easy to apply and remove. It stimulates blood circulation, detoxifies, exfoliates dead skin cells and reduces the appearance of wrinkles, leaving the skin soft, smooth and invigorated.

It produces erythema (local skin warming), accelerates physiological processes and increases cell regeneration in surrounding tissues, improving skin elasticity and overall complexion. It is an excellent choice of clay for ageing skin, due to its soft but stimulating and rejuvenating effect.

6.8. Green Clays

Green Clays - Illite and Montmorillonite
Green clays are mostly of sedimentary origin, resulting from sedimentation and weathering of volcanic ashes which are found near ancient volcanoes, 20-50 meters below the ground surface. Green clays are rich in magnesium and several trace elements. They are very popular in the cosmetic and beauty industry. There are two types of green clay used - montmorillonite and illite.

I have come across many sites selling green clay as such, without specifying whether it is montmorillonite or illite. I think that since these two clays have differences in their chemical make-up and structure which affects their physical properties, they need to be described separately.

There are two types of green clay used in natural medicine - montmorillonite and illite. Montmorillonite is part of the smectite group of clays and is named after a French region Montmorillon. Illite is named after the state Illinois, USA, where it was first identified in 1937. Both clays take equally important places in the restoration and maintenance of health. However, as mentioned earlier, there are certain differences.

The sorptive properties of green montmorillonite are less than those of illite, but its remineralisation properties are very high - 70%. The cationic exchange capacity of the French green montmorillonite is many times higher than that of the green illite.

Both illite and montmorillonite clays absorb water. However, the montmorillonite clay is called 'the swelling' type, while illite clays are called 'non-swelling'. The illite clays have a highly porous crystal structure, so water gets inside the crystals, which makes the clay so sorbent (just like a sponge).

With montmorillonite, on the other hand, water gets between the flat layers in the clay particles, which make the layers move apart, causing the 'swelling' effect (similar to rising puff pastry when baked). It is between those layers that cation exchange happens when montmorillonite clay is hydrated.

6.9. Green Montmorillonite Clay

Green montmorillonite clay is one of the most popular clays used in cosmetics and healing. It contains a variety of minerals and salts, including calcium, potassium, dolomite, magnesium, silica, manganese, phosphorous, silicon, copper, and selenium. These elements are essential in producing body enzymes which enhance the production of enzymes in all living organisms.

Green clay is greyish green. Its colour is due to the presence of ferrous and magnesium ions. Green Montmorillonite clay is the best clay for oily skin since it reduces sebum production acting as a wonderful absorbent and exfoliator.

It is rich in important minerals and phytonutrients and is one of the most commonly used therapeutic clays. It is a great choice for face masks, body wraps, compresses, baths, poultices and other procedures. It is also excellent for intestinal cleansing programmes.

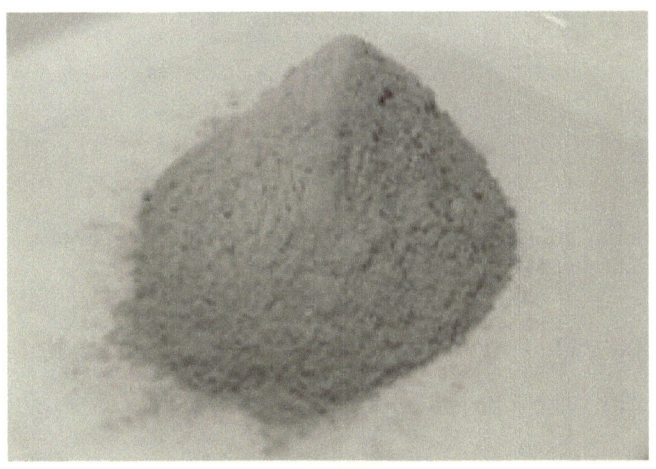

Green montmorillonite is a swelling type of clay absorbing water at the 1:1 rate. This means that its crystalline structure can shift outwards when hydrated with water, increasing its active surface. So the clay creates spaces for water between its layers. Recent research indicates that French Green clay can bind mycotoxins in the digestive system of animals, as well as several bacteria in-vitro.

"In experiments, the clay killed up to 99 per cent of superbug colonies within 24 hours. Control samples of MRSA (methicillin-resistant Staphylococcus aureus) grew 45-fold in the same period. The clay has a similar effect on other deadly bacteria tested, including salmonella, E. coli, and a flesh-eating disease called Buruli, a relative of leprosy which disfigures children across central and western Africa. It has been classed as "an emerging public health threat" by the World Health Organization (WHO)."

The effectiveness of the green clays, which are mostly made of minerals called smectite and illite, was first demonstrated by Line Brunet de Courssou, a French doctor fighting Buruli at clinics in Ivory Coast and Guinea." (Source: independent.co.uk/life-style/health-and-families/health-news/french-muck-is-this-the-new-penicillin-5328853.html)

A German scientist once described bactericidal properties of clay: "The curative properties of clay are founded in its special physical characteristics, above all in the distribution of its minute particles. Individual clay particles are smaller than many bacteria.

If infected mucous membranes are more or less flooded with clay, the bacteria are surrounded by clay particles and are thus separated from their source of nourishment and become embedded in the inorganic material. Growth and the survivability of the bacteria are thus halted almost instantaneously, and from this explained strikingly speedy abatement of the symptoms of infection and/or symptoms of poisoning in acute infectious diseases of the alimentary canal." Julius Stumpf, Bolus fur medizinische Anwenduno Darmstadt, 1916, p. 19.

Green montmorillonite clay is closely related to bentonite clay - they belong to the same group of smectite clays. It is rich in magnesium, iron, manganese, calcium, silica and other macro and microelements. It speeds up blood circulation and regeneration of tissues and helps to bind and take out of the body harmful free radicals.

Due to its high ion exchange capacity, green montmorillonite clay is a superb detoxification product. Its detoxifying properties are explained by 2 main factors:

1. Its negative cumulative ionic charge which helps to attract and bind positively charged toxic waste and eliminate it out of the body.
2. Its ability to swell in water and expand due to its high montmorillonite content. This expansion means a larger sorptive area which allows the clay particles to attract a much higher percentage of toxins than it would otherwise.

Green montmorillonite clay acts like a sponge, attracting water and toxins not only to its negatively charged surface but also inside numerous canals, 'trapping' them there via ionic exchange process. The body gets the 'good' mineral from the clay in return.

In the beauty industry, this clay is a great cleanser which will benefit most skin types, especially when treating oily and congested skin.

6.10. Green Illite Clay

Green illite clay is efficient at drawing oils and toxins from the skin. It is a non-swelling clay. It is sometimes called 'marine clay' because the quarries are based around ancient marine beds. This explains a rich mineral content of illite clay. It has a better absorption ability than montmorillonite. Its sorptive properties give it a very powerful drying and detoxifying effect. With its very high sorption capacity, illite acts like a magnet for toxins, so it is the greatest detoxifying remedy available in nature.

Green Illite clay is a superb detoxification product. Its detoxifying properties are explained by 2 main factors:

1. Its sorptive capacity is very high, so it draws toxins out of the body very effectively.
2. Its negative cumulative ionic charge which helps to attract and bind positively charged toxic waste and eliminate it out of the body.

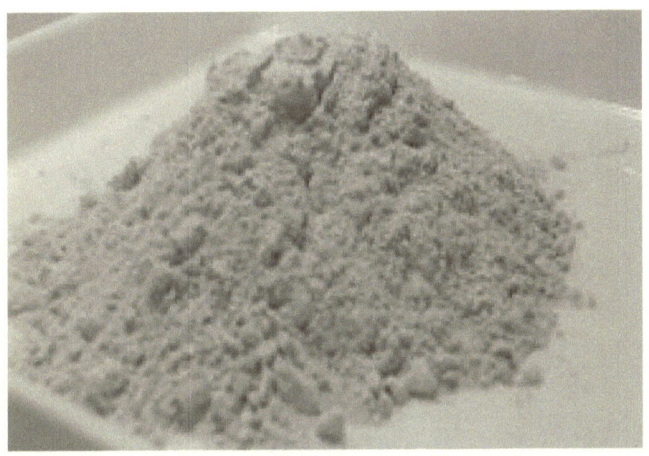

French green illite clay acts like a sponge, attracting water and toxins not only to its negatively charged surface but also inside the numerous canals in its crystalline structure.

Both clays have similar properties, with one clay detoxifying the body due to its higher sorption capacity (illite), and the other due to its ability to expand and attract negatively charged ions. Green Illite is favoured by health practitioners worldwide.

Both green clays contain such elements as silica, magnesium, calcium, iron, potassium, cobalt, manganese, zinc, selenium, copper, aluminium, phosphorous, sodium, as well as others.

6.11. Rhassoul Clay

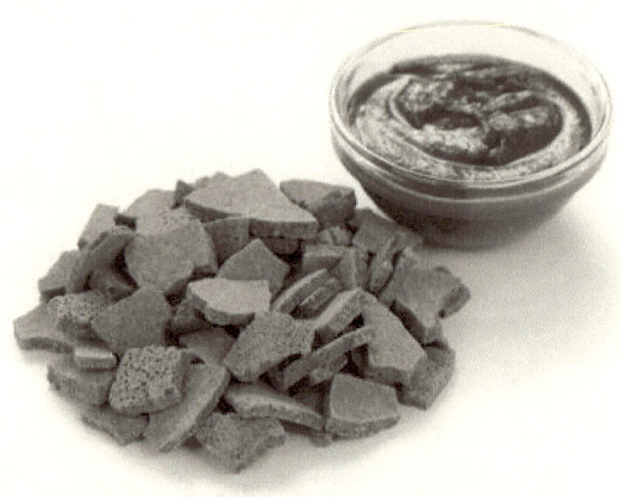

Rhassoul (Ghassoul, Maroc) clay is part of the smectite (swelling) group of clay minerals. It is mineral-rich, reddish-brown ancient clay which comes from the Atlas Mountains of Morocco. It has been traditionally used in Morocco and Egypt as soap, shampoo and skin conditioner. Rhassoul clay is truly exquisite and is different from other clays due to its unique composition, excellent ability to adsorb oils and impurities.

It is very high in trace elements such as silica, magnesium, iron, calcium, potassium and sodium. Because of the high mineral content, astringent and absorption properties, Rhassoul clay is wonderful and effective clay for cleansing, detoxification, and general skincare treatments.

It has been shown to improve skin elasticity, clear clogged pores, remove dead skin, excessive oil from skin, stimulate circulation, nourish and hydrate the skin. Rhassoul clay can be used in soap-making, facial masks, body wraps, clay packs, shampoos, and conditioners. It is used by the best spas around the world and is highly regarded in the beauty industry. It is suitable for normal and oily skin.

6.12. Yellow Illite Clay

Yellow illite clay has a soft yellow colour and velvety texture. It is very similar to green illite in its therapeutic and cosmetic properties and uses. Its colour is due to a high level of iron oxide.

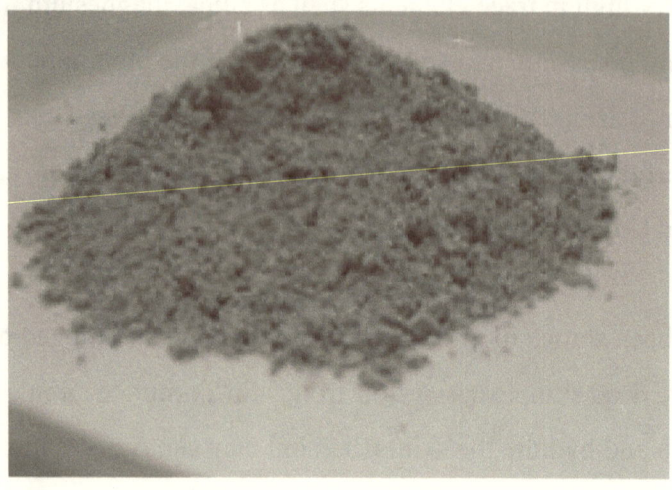

Illite is found in certain regions in the North of France and the Atlantic basin, in the areas abundant in red clays. It is highly sorbent and has a relatively low cation exchange rate.

It has a beautiful, soft velvety texture and is most suitable for ageing, sallow, blemished skin types. It is also great for sensitive oily acne-prone skin. This clay is great as a colour agent in cosmetics and soap making.

6.13. Red Illite Clay

Red illite clay is similar in properties to green and other illite clays. Its main property is high sorptive capacity - similar to other illite clays. The only difference is its colouring which is explained by a higher presence of iron oxide.

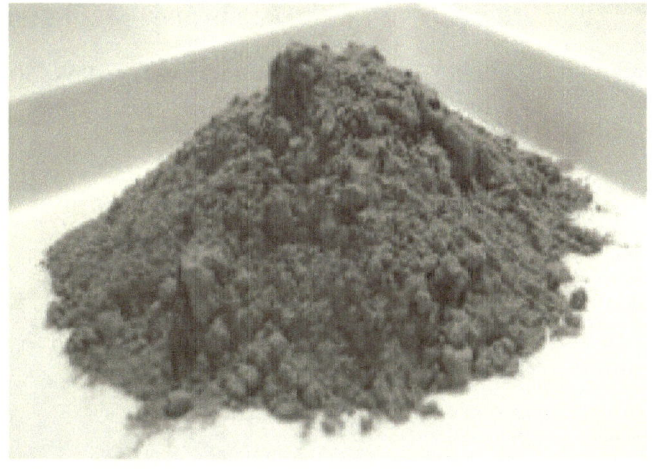

Red illite clay is used mainly in the beauty industry and cosmetics production, for its toning, humidifying effect on the skin. It revives pale, sallow, ageing skin. It also purifies congested, acne-prone skin types. This clay is great at treating broken capillaries and thread veins. It improves blood circulation and makes the skin look radiant, hydrated, reducing the appearance of wrinkles.

6.14. Pink Illite Clay

French pink illite is not a type of clay which is naturally mined. It is a mix of two French clays - white kaolin and red illite and is mainly used in the beauty and cosmetics industry thanks to its soft, soothing, toning action on the skin.

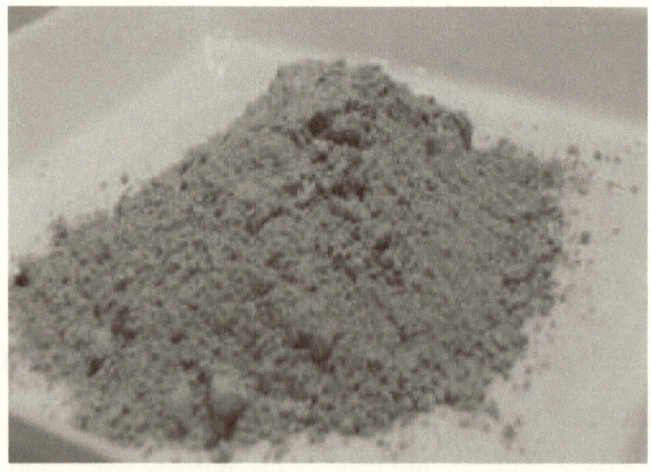

It is suitable for all skin types, but especially for mature skin, prone to wrinkle formation and flushing. Sensitive, fragile skin types also benefit from the use of French pink illite clay. It is great for conditions where gentle drying action is required.

6.15. White Kaolin Clay

White white kaolin clay is the most abundant mineral in the kaolinite group. It is also known as China clay or white cosmetic clay.

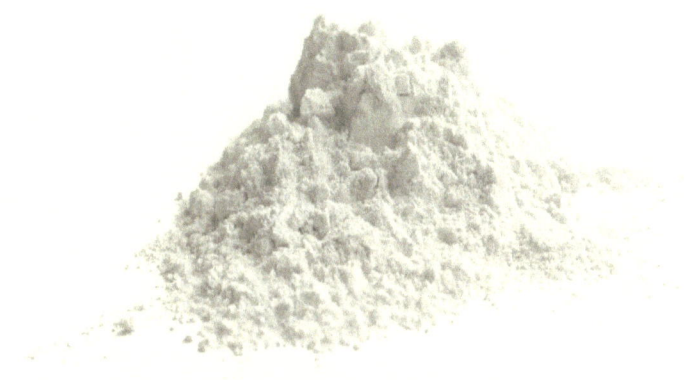

It owes its colour to a high concentration of aluminium (in a bound form, like with all clays). It is the most used clay in cosmetics. It is an essential ingredient in the manufacturing of cosmetics - soaps, scrubs, poultices, body and face powders. It is also used as a fixative in the perfume industry.

It is the mildest of all the cosmetic clays and Its action on the skin is very gentle, so it can be used on most sensitive skin types. It adsorbs impurities from the skin without removing any natural oils. It helps to stimulate circulation in the skin, while gently exfoliating and cleansing it. Its adsorption effect is minimal, so it does not draw oils from the skin, so it can be used on dry and sensitive skin.

7. Toxins & Sources of Toxicity

To fully understand the importance of detoxification, we need to learn what toxins can be found in the environment surrounding us, water, air, food, products we use, how they get into the living organism, and what effect they have on us. Toxins are defined by most dictionaries as poisonous substances produced by plants, bacteria, viruses or fungi, algae, plants, insects and animals.

A toxin is a poisonous substance produced within living cells or organisms; synthetic substances created by artificial processes are thus excluded. The term was first used by organic chemist Ludwig Brieger (1849–1919). Toxins can be small molecules, peptides, or proteins that are capable of causing disease on contact with or absorption by body tissues interacting with biological macromolecules such as enzymes or cellular receptors. Toxins vary greatly in their severity, ranging from usually minor and acute (as in a bee sting) to almost immediately deadly (as in botulinum toxin)." (Source: en.wikipedia.org/wiki/Toxin)

Toxins can be divided into several groups:

- Bacteria, viruses, fungi, protozoa

- Naturally occurring toxins (e.g. aflatoxins, mould, glycoalkaloids in green potatoes, algal toxins in shellfish, etc.)
- Inorganic toxins: heavy/radioactive metals, excessive amounts of 'good' minerals in the body
- Man-made toxins: pesticides, fertilisers, E-numbers, additives, artificially created dies and preservatives in food and cosmetics, medicines and medical procedures (Medicines can have numerous side-effects aiming to treat a condition but disrupting many body organs and processes in the meantime – e.g. chemotherapy drugs, radiotherapy procedures).

The problem with toxins is that most of them do not enter the body suddenly (unless it is a case of acute poisoning), but accumulate in it over many years. Toxic overload is responsible for many health problems we suffer from today. Toxins destroy our bodies without us knowing it.

We get sick at various stages in our lives. We think that the flu that has immobilised us for a couple of weeks is what is meant to happen when we are around people carrying a virus. How can we avoid it if everyone around us is sneezing! We accept that we will probably become sick once the epidemic starts. But not everyone catches flu during flu epidemics. Some of us are more at risk than others. Body toxicity undermines our immune system, making us less resistant to infection.

A similar picture can be observed with other diseases. Some of us become victims of heart disease, diabetes, cancer while others don't. Scientists have discovered that our genetic make-up is only 5% responsible for our predisposition to some of these illnesses. The rest 95% is due to the environmental factors, lifestyle, nutrition and our response to life situations.

The body has vast coping resources which are given to us by nature. Of course, genetic disorders exist and do make people ill. Some people are born with them. But in the vast majority of cases, our conditions are acquired as a result of a prolonged attack by environmental toxins which come from medicines, dental fillings, water and food contaminants, substance abuse, poor lifestyle and nutrition, emotional issues and other similar things. Unborn children are not safe either – a mother's exposure to these factors impacts the child in her womb without mercy. These factors can also trigger any genetic predisposition we have to an illness.

The two major killers of out times – heart disease and cancer – have much to do not only with our unhealthy lifestyle, nutrition and stress but also with the toxins that invade our bodies. The same can be said about fertility problems, genetic mutations, birth defects, child cancers and many other diseases.

7.1. Biological Toxins

These include poisonous substances produced by bacteria, viruses, fungi, algae, animals, insects and plants. They are normally called "biotoxins". These are further subdivided into groups, depending on their origin. There is a group of toxins which is produced by animals, fish, sea inhabitants and insects - these are called "zoo-toxins". These toxins are either used for protection or aggression.

Here is a list of most common biotoxins:

- Cyanotoxins, produced by cyanobacteria
- Photo-toxins - cause severe photosensitivity (normally zoo-toxins)
- Hemotoxins - attack red blood cells (normally zoo-toxins)
- Necrotoxins - cause necrosis of tissues they are in contact with (normally zoo-toxins)

- Neurotoxins - attack nervous system (normally zoo-toxins)
- Cytotoxins - attack individual cells (normally zoo-toxins)
- Mycotoxins - produced by fungi, normally affecting grains and other foods.
- Aflatoxins - found in food, water, environment.

Toxins naturally occurring in foods (biological origin)

Most foods contain varying amounts of toxins which are minute and are not dangerous to health. However, there are foods which contain a high level of toxins, and these foods fall under strict supervision and regulation by the Food Standards Agency (UK) or FDA (USA).

Some substances only affect some people and not others, due to the inability of the body to metabolise the substances - for example, lactose, gluten, certain sugars, etc. This results in various health problems, such as autoimmune disorder. Others are dangerous to all living organisms. Here is a list of some of the toxins which naturally occur in foods:

- **Cyanogenic glycosides** - these are found in cassava and unprocessed bamboo shoots. Correct preparation reduces the amount of these toxins and makes these food products safe to eat.

- **Amygdalin** - cyanogenic glycoside contained in fruit seeds and stones - "Apple and pear seeds and the inner stony pit (kernel) of apricots and peaches contain a naturally occurring substance called amygdalin which is a cyanogenic glycoside. Amygdalin can release hydrogen cyanide in the stomach causing discomfort or illness. It can sometimes be fatal." (Source: foodsafety.asn.au/natural-toxins-in-food)

- **Ipomeamarone** - a toxin encountered in sweet potato - kumara, especially if it is damaged. Damaged parts of kumara need to be discarded before cooking, and if it tastes bitter after cooking.

- **Furocoumarins** - encountered in parsnips, especially damaged parts, and the peel. Peeling, cleaning parsnips of any damaged parts and cooking reduces the number of toxins.

- **Glycoalkaloids** - occur in potatoes. The level rises dramatically in sprouted, stressed potatoes, or the ones exposed to light and turned green as a result. Glycoalkaloids are highly poisonous and do not get destroyed during cooking, so it's important to discard sprouted or green potatoes.

- **Alcohol** - natural toxin. The liver goes under a lot of stress processing alcohol, so its intake should be limited, especially by pregnant women.
- **Mushrooms** - some mushrooms are very toxic and can lead to death if consumed. Avoid a mushroom if you don't know what species it is.
- Certain types of **fish and seafood** can be very toxic, so should be avoided. Some fish contains a large amount of **mercury** - e.g. shark, swordfish, and their consumption should be strictly limited.
- **Lectins** - highly toxic substances contained in beans. Red kidney beans have an especially high concentration of them, so correct cooking is important.
- **Cucurbitacins** - found in zucchini. These toxins give the vegetable a bitter taste. Do not eat zucchini which has a bitter taste and unpleasant smell.
- **Selenium in the grain** - can accumulate naturally due to microbial activity. This means that people consuming grains can have selenium toxicity which is a danger to health.
- **Goitrogens** - toxins affecting the thyroid function. Foods such as spinach, cassava, peanuts, soybeans, strawberries, sweet potatoes, peaches, pears, and vegetables in the *Brassica* genu contain these toxins. It is especially

common in uncooked broccoli, Brussels sprouts, cabbage, canola, cauliflower, mustard greens, radishes, and rapeseed.

7.2. Environmental Toxins

These are mostly man-made synthetic substances which become toxic to humans and animals when they enter the body in quantities which are either dangerous or have a potential to accumulate and change bodily functions. Such toxins include fertilisers, pesticides, certain substances from plastics, domestic products, cosmetic ingredients, food and drink additives and preservatives, medicines, alcohol, tobacco, fuel and products resulting from its use, and more.

When these substances enter the body in dangerous levels or accumulate in it over a while, they can cause a lot of damage. This is not to scare you or say that what you eat/drink is dangerous.

Air and water pollutants which present danger to health

These include industrial fumes, pesticides, dioxins, pharmaceutical hormones, benzene, phthalate DEHP, organic solvents, DDT, vinyl chloride, aromatic amines, Polycyclic Aromatic Hydrocarbons (PAHs), Poly-chlorinated Biphenyls (PCBs), tobacco smoke, non-ionising radiation among many others.

Here is a list of some of environmental toxins and pollutants:

- **Hydraulic fracturing (fracking)** - a process which is used in the production of oil and gas. Fracking fluids can contain chemicals linked to breast cancer, including known and suspected **carcinogens** such as **benzene** and **toluene**, and endocrine-disrupting compounds such as the phthalate DEHP. Evidence is beginning to emerge that these chemicals may contaminate underground water sources.

- **Dioxin** - found in both water and air, as a result of breaking down of chlorine. Dioxins are known human carcinogens and endocrine disruptors. One dioxin has been classified by the International Agency for Research on Cancer (IARC) and the Environmental Protection Agency (EPA) as a known human carcinogen.

- **Endocrine disruptors from wastewater** - these include compounds found in the hormone replacement medications and contraceptives, as well as personal care products. They cannot be completely removed from wastewater, so a percentage end up in tap water.

- **Organic solvents** - chemicals which include chlorinated and other solvents, such as methylene chloride, trichloroethylene and formaldehyde. Sources of exposure include outdoor and indoor air pollution, waste incineration, cleaning products and some cosmetics. They are also used in the manufacture of computer parts.

- **Pesticides** - Many pesticides, including herbicides and other pest-killing poisons, have been labelled as human or animal carcinogens. A 2006 report demonstrated that lifetime use of residential pesticides may be associated with an increase in risk for breast cancer. Studies have found that many of these chemicals are present in water supplies, as well as in samples of air and dust from homes.

- **1,3-butadiene** - present in tobacco smoke. It is also used in the manufacture of some rubber products and fungicides. The main route of exposure is inhalation. Found to be a carcinogen.

- **Aromatic amines** - found in tobacco smoke, and are a by-product of plastic manufacturing and chemical industries. "One aromatic amine is known to cause mammary tumors in rodents. They can also have direct effects on cell division, which may enhance the development of tumours.

- **Vinyl chloride** - found in wastewater as a result of the production of PVC (polyvinyl chloride), in the air near hazardous waste sites, and tobacco smoke. Vinyl chloride was one of the first chemicals designated as a known human carcinogen by the National Toxicology Program (NTP). It has also been linked to increased mortality from breast cancer among workers involved in its manufacture.

- **Polycyclic aromatic hydrocarbons (PAHs)** - by-products of combustion, from sources as varied as coal burners, diesel engines, grilled meats and cigarettes. PAH residues are often found in the air and house dust. Exposure is primarily through inhalation. They have been shown to increase the risk of breast cancer.

- **Light at night (LAN)** - is an environmental pollutant which disrupts the production of melatonin - the sleep hormone with anti-cancer properties. Research suggests a link between night-shift work and increased risk of breast cancer, possibly through this melatonin-LAN pathway.

- **Non-Ionising Radiation** - Electromagnetic waves are a type of non-ionizing radiation. They are produced by cell phones, wireless networking, radio towers, computers and electric lighting. The International Agency for Research on Cancer (IARC) has classified electromagnetic fields as possible human carcinogens, but consensus has been difficult to reach.

- **Tobacco smoke** - Tobacco smoke contains polycyclic aromatic hydrocarbons (PAHs), which may explain a potential link between increased breast cancer risk and both active and passive smoke inhalation. Tobacco smoke contains hundreds of other chemicals, including three known human carcinogens. A recent study found that both active and passive smoke inhalation increase the risk of breast cancer in pre-menopausal women.

- **Benzene** - one of the highest volume petrochemical solvents currently in production, and global production rates are expected to continue to grow. It has been designated as a known human carcinogen. Exposure comes from inhaling gas fumes, automobile exhaust and tobacco smoke. Benzene poses a serious hazard for people exposed through manufacturing and refining industries.

- **Polychlorinated Biphenyls (PCBs)** - banned in 1976, but according to the statistics, as many as two-thirds of all insulation fluids, plastics, adhesives, paper, inks, paints and other products containing PCB manufactured before the ban remain in daily use. One type of PCB acts like an estrogen; a second, like an anti-estrogen; and a third appears not to be hormonally active. Therefore, most studies look at total PCB levels.

- The source for this information was a website formerly known under the URL breastcancerfund.org, currently bcpp.org. The website and information available on it have changed since I wrote this book. However, other sources confirm the information above.

- Following is a list of most common household hazards which can be toxic at certain levels - compiled based on the Top 10 Common Household Toxins (Source: content.time.com/time/specials/packages/article/0,28804,1 976909_1976895,00.html):

- **Bisphenol A (BPA)** - found in plastics food packaging, bottles, baby bottles. There is concern about the brain and behavioural effects of bisphenol on fetuses and young children at current exposure levels.

- **Oxybenzone** - a chemical used in cosmetic products such as lip balm, moisturisers, sunscreen lotion. Its use has been linked to low birth rate in babies and hormone disruption.

- **Fluoride** - a form of basic element fluorine found in water and toothpaste. It is neurotoxic and carcinogenic. The American Dental Association advises against its use in children under 2 years old. However, it is still being added to water supplies worldwide.

- **Parabens** - cosmetic preservatives, found in shaving products, hair care products, moisturisers. Causes hormone disruption and cancer in animals. Current exposure is deemed safe, but paraben-free products are available.

- **Phthalates** - give plastics resilience and flexibility. They are found in food packaging, detergents, shampoos, toys, shower curtains, raincoats, shower curtains, vinyl flooring. These are linked to low sperm count, reproductive abnormalities, liver cancer in humans.

- **Butylated hydroxyanisole (BHA)** - added to oils, snack foods, chewing gum, diaper cream. May lead to cancer.

- **Perfluorooctanoic acid (PFOA)** - a component in Teflon (non-stick coating used in pans, frying pans and other utensils). Has been found to cause hormone disruption and reproductive abnormalities, as well as cancer. If you have to use it, avoid heating empty utensils to high temperatures.

- **Perchlorate** - antioxidant in rocket fuel. Found in drinking water, some vegetables, soil. Causes disruption of the thyroid function.

- **Decabromodiphenyl ether (DECA)** - flame retardant. Used in carpets, household goods, electronics. Causes permanent learning and memory deficiencies, hearing defects, decreased sperm count.

- **Asbestos** - a natural fibrous mineral. Found in housing insulation, toys, drywall and artificial fireplace logs. Causes mesothelioma which is fatal cancer. It is not always labelled by the manufacturers.

- **Aflatoxins** - The toxins - the researcher said - are in the water, soil and airborne, the fungi that produce them are an olive green mould that can be found in refrigerators, besides they are very resistant to high temperatures. "Mexican scientists identified and quantified the number of aflatoxins (carcinogenic) in food such as corn tortilla, rice, chilli pepper, processed sauces, chicken breast and eggs, and revealed its relationship with cervical and liver cancer in humans… This research is the first in the world to report that cervical cancer can also be caused by ingesting aflatoxin-contaminated food. This carcinogenic has also been detected as a trigger of colorectal, pancreatic, breast and lung cancer." (Source: sciencedaily.com/releases/2013/09/130930161927.htm)

7.3. Heavy Metals

There is a debate as to what constitutes a heavy metal. Some use the atomic weight, while others base the name of the element valency (ability to bind other chemical elements). The majority of researchers who write about heavy metal toxicity define any metal which is dangerous to human health in small amounts as heavy. Heavy metal toxicity can arise from acute or prolonged exposure to certain substances which contain heavy metals.

Here is a detailed reference table of the symptoms caused by heavy metal toxicity: emedicine.medscape.com/article/814960-overview.

Many of the elements which can be considered heavy metals have no known benefits to humans. Such elements include lead, mercury, cadmium and many others. However, other metals are essential to biochemical processes. For example, zinc takes part in various enzymatic reactions, vitamin B-12 includes cobalt as part of it, and haemoglobin contains iron. Copper, manganese, selenium, chromium, and molybdenum are all trace elements, which play an important role in the human body. Other metals are used therapeutically in medicine. They include aluminium, bismuth, gold, gallium, lithium, and silver. Any of these elements may damage the body if taken in excessive amounts or if natural mechanisms of elimination are impaired.

Symptoms of heavy metal toxicity vary depending on the heavy metal involved, total dose absorbed, and whether the exposure is acute or chronic. The age of the person can also influence toxicity. For example, young children are more prone to the effects of lead exposure because they absorb several times of the total ingested amount compared with adults and because their brain is still growing and developing, so has more plasticity. Even brief exposures may influence developmental processes. The route of exposure is also important. Elemental mercury is relatively inert in the gastrointestinal tract and also poorly absorbed through intact skin. However, if inhaled or injected, elemental mercury may have disastrous effects.

Various toxins affect the body in different ways. Some of the symptoms can be similar, and it may be very difficult to diagnose the reason for a certain symptom unless there is a strong obvious link to the cause.

Toxin exposure can cause a variety of symptoms, starting from mild discomfort, leading to more serious symptoms, such as vomiting, diarrhoea, loss of consciousness, mental retardation, chronic diseases, cancer, and even death. Many of the symptoms have been covered when describing the toxins. For information on the symptoms of heavy metal toxicity, see the table above.

Here is a list of symptoms resulting from heavy metal toxicity:

- **Selenium** - exposure to high doses can cause selenosis which can cause hair loss, nail brittleness, and neurological abnormalities (numbness in the extremities). "Symptoms of selenosis include a garlic odour on the breath, gastrointestinal disorders, hair loss, sloughing of nails, fatigue, irritability, and neurological damage. Extreme cases of selenosis can result in cirrhosis of the liver, pulmonary oedema, and death." (Source: en.wikipedia.org/wiki/Selenium#Toxicity)

- **Beryllium** - exposure to high doses can cause chronic beryllium disease, which may result in breathing difficulties, coughing, chest pain.

- **Mercury** - exposure to it can cause damage to the central nervous system and kidneys. "Mercury poisoning can result in several diseases, including acrodynia (pink disease), Hunter-Russell syndrome, and Minamata disease. Symptoms typically include sensory impairment (vision, hearing, speech), disturbed sensation and a lack of coordination. The type and degree of symptoms exhibited depend upon the individual toxin, the dose, and the method and duration of exposure." (Source: en.wikipedia.org/wiki/Mercury_poisoning).

- **Chromium (IV)** - exposure can cause strong allergic reaction linked to Asthmatic Bronchitis and DNA damage. "After it reaches the bloodstream, it damages the kidneys, the liver and blood cells through oxidation reactions. Hemolysis, renal and liver failure are the results of these damages." (Source: en.wikipedia.org/wiki/Chromium_toxicity)

- **Arsenic** - long term exposure can cause lung cancer, skin disease, nerve damage. "Symptoms of arsenic poisoning begin with headaches, confusion, severe diarrhoea, and drowsiness. As the poisoning develops, convulsions and changes in fingernail pigmentation called leukonychia striata may occur. When the poisoning becomes acute, symptoms may include diarrhoea, vomiting, blood in the urine, cramping muscles, hair loss, stomach pain, and more convulsions. The organs of the body that are usually affected by arsenic poisoning are the lungs, skin, kidneys, and liver." (Source: en.wikipedia.org/wiki/Arsenic_poisoning)

- **Lead** - exposure to it can cause nervous system, kidney damage, blood disorders, cancer and foetal abnormalities. Children are especially vulnerable. "Lead interferes with a variety of body processes and is toxic to many organs and tissues including the heart, bones, intestines, kidneys, and reproductive and nervous systems. It interferes with the development of the nervous system and is therefore particularly toxic to children, causing potentially permanent learning and behaviour disorders. Symptoms include abdominal pain, confusion, headache, anaemia, irritability, and in severe cases seizures, coma, and death." Source: en.wikipedia.org/wiki/Lead_poisoning

Symptoms also include nausea, vomiting, headaches, seizures, encephalopathy, anaemia, abdominal pain, nephropathy, foot-drop, wrist-drop.

- **Barium** - exposure may lead to brain swelling, high blood pressure, damage to heart, liver and spleen.
- **Bismuth** - renal failure, acute tubular necrosis.

- **Cadmium** - long term exposure can cause kidney and liver damage, lung cancer, osteomalacia, or even death. Cadmium is contained in cigarette smoke and car fumes. It is also a well-known carcinogen.

- **Cobalt** - beer drinker's (dilated) cardiomyopathy, pneumoconiosis, goitre.

- **Copper** - irritation of GI tract, irritation, vineyard sprayer's lung (when inhaled), hepatic degeneration.

- **Iron** - vomiting, GI haemorrhage, cardiac depression, metabolic acidosis, hepatic cirrhosis.

- **Manganese** - Parkinson-like syndrome, respiratory problems, neuropsychiatric disorders.

- **Nickel** - dermatitis, myocarditis, encephalopathy, occupational pulmonary fibrosis (inhaled), low sperm count, tumours in the nasal area and pharynx.

- **Selenium** - caustic burns, pneumonitis, hypotension, brittle nails and hair, red skin, hemiplegia.

- **Silver (high doses)** - haemorrhage, bone marrow suppression, pulmonary oedema, hepato-renal necrosis, blue-grey discolouration of the skin & nails.

- **Thallium** - early symptoms include vomiting, diarrhoea, painful neuropathy, coma, autonomic instability. Late symptoms: residual neurologic symptoms, alopecia (hair loss).

- **Zinc** - vomiting, diarrhoea, abdominal pain, copper deficiency, anaemia, neurologic degeneration, osteoporosis.

Mercury is one of the most abundant and most toxic substances we are exposed to. Chronic exposure to mercury produces neurological, physical and psychological/ psychiatric symptoms. Physical symptoms include reduced immunity leading to increased exposure to bacterial, viral and fungal infections, tumours (including various cancers), fatigue (including Chronic Fatigue Syndrome), gingivitis and allergic reactions.

"Other symptoms may include: headache, unsteady gait, numbness and pain in the extremities, muscular weakness, paraesthesias, drowsiness, slurring of words, slight stammering, difficulty in pronunciation of words, oedema, metallic taste, loosened teeth, increased salivation, loss of weight, hair loss, nausea, constipation, diarrhoea, other gastrointestinal disturbances, difficulty in breathing..." (Source: algonet.se/~leif/AmFAQk02.html#GENERAL)

Psychological/ psychiatric symptoms include irritability, stress intolerance, increased sensitivity to light and sound, outbursts of temper, resentment of criticism, shyness, anxiety, depression, insomnia, indecision, fatigue, memory loss, etc.

Other effects of mercury include:

- Reduced effectiveness of antibiotics
- Reduction in levels of neurotransmitters, including serotonin. This can lead to the development of depression, addictions, anxiety, anger.
- Depressed heart function
- Causes the development of cancer cells
- Slowing down of the endocrine function
- May cause damage to kidney cells
- Reduction of blood supply to the foetus
- Development of learning disabilities in young children

- Damage to the immune system, resulting in allergies, autoimmune diseases, asthma.

Much of mercury gets into the body from mercury amalgam fillings (50% of mercury), childhood vaccines, fish, seafood, paint. Mercury fillings are especially dangerous, since they gradually leak, and mercury gets deposited in the brain, spinal cord and nerve tissue causing them irreversible damage. "In deceased adult humans, there is a correlation, on a group level, between the amount of Hg in the brain and the number of amalgam-fillings ". Nylander 1987, Weiner 1993 (Source: algonet.se/%7Eleif/yfWEI93a.html).

Research has shown that "Hg (mercury) from dental amalgam will appear in maternal and fetal blood and amniotic fluid within 2 days after placement of amalgam tooth restorations." (Am J Physiol 258:R939-R945 (1990)). This study demonstrates that mercury in fillings passes from a pregnant mother to the foetus.

Acrodynia (the Pink Disease) is a result of mercury intoxication. "The names Acrodynia / Pink Disease point in the direction of something specific and almost obligatory in this form of Hg-intoxication; pink peeling skin and extreme pain at/in distal extremities. Profuse sweating is a common symptom. Other symptoms can be low-grade intermittent fever as well as hypertonia and tachycardia. Any of the symptoms described in chronic mercury intoxication... can be present. It seems to mainly affect younger children, but can affect adults as well." (Source: algonet.se – the website is no longer online).

Children are much more vulnerable as far as mercury and other heavy metal toxicity are concerned since their tissues are more permeable and brains are more plastic, so even brief exposure can cause disastrous developmental consequences. Also, they absorb several times the percentage of ingested mercury compared to adults. So mercury toxicity in children is therefore much more dangerous.

Another source of mercury poisoning is thimerosal. This is what FDA says about thimerosal in vaccines on its website: "Thimerosal is a mercury-containing organic compound (an organomercurial). Since the 1930s, it has been widely used as a preservative in many biological and drug products, including many vaccines, to help prevent potentially life-threatening contamination with harmful microbes.

Over the past several years, because of increasing awareness of the theoretical potential for neurotoxicity of even low levels of organomercurials and because of the increased number of thimerosal-containing vaccines that had been added to the infant immunization schedule, concerns about the use of thimerosal in vaccines and other products have been raised. Indeed, because of these concerns, the Food and Drug Administration has worked with and continues to work with, vaccine manufacturers to reduce or eliminate thimerosal from vaccines." (Source: fda.gov/BiologicsBloodVaccines/SafetyAvailability/VaccineSafet y/UCM096228)

Two types of mercury can be deposited in the body – organic and inorganic. Organic mercury is many times more dangerous since it can easily penetrate cell walls, get absorbed by fatty tissues and by nerve and brain cells. Organic mercury forms from inorganic one by attaching itself to organic molecules CH3 called a "methyl group", and is potentially much more destructive to the body cells. The mercury from fish is organic mercury with the chemical formula CH3HgCH3.

Another form of organic mercury gets formed in the colon, influenced by the H2S gas produced by the Candida fungus and the bad bacteria and the enzyme Thiolmethyl Transferase (THT). This way any inorganic mercury which has been deposited in the body for years mixes up with the organic molecules and becomes organic. Methyl mercury attacks the cerebellum responsible for coordinating voluntary movements and destroys the personality.

Since bad bacteria and fungi cause fermentation of the food and the production of the H2S gas, an unhealthy gut contributes to the conversion of inorganic mercury into the organic one. So possibly the best way of getting rid of mercury is to cleanse one's gut, and clays are the best natural choice for it.

In her lecture, Dr Dietrich Klinghardt describes how mercury affects the body organs and tissues:

"From a scientific point of view, there is no more "controversy" about the ill health effects of the metals contained in and released by the typical dental amalgam fillings. The sheep and monkey studies conducted at the University of Calgary, Canada-' under the guidance of Dr. Murray Vimy DDS-showed that radioactively labelled mercury released from freshly and correctly placed amalgam fillings (in a monkey study) appeared quickly in the kidneys, brain and wall of the intestines.
Through its affinity for sulfhydryl-groups, mercury bonds very firmly to structures in the nervous system. Other studies showed that mercury is taken up in the periphery by all nerve endings (i.e. the hypoglossal nerve of the tongue, the autonomic nerves of the

lung or intestinal wall and connective tissue) and rapidly transported inside the axon of the nerves (axonal transport) to the spinal cord and brainstem.

On its way from the periphery to the brain, mercury immobilizes the enzyme that is essential for "making" tubulin. Tubulin forms tubular structures within each nerve, along which the nerve-cell transports metabolic waste from the nerve cell into the periphery and along which the nutrients required by the nerve cell are transported from the periphery to the cell.

Once mercury has travelled up the axon, the nerve cell is impaired in its ability to detoxify itself and in its ability to nurture itself. The cell becomes toxic and dies - or lives in a state of chronic malnutrition. The mercury that has entered the nerve cell can no longer be excreted in the normal axonal transport routes (some can exit through the $Ca++$ and $Na+-$ channels) and begins to exert its more well-known ill-effects on the mitochondria, nucleus and other organelles of the cell. A multitude of illnesses, usually associated with neurological symptoms, result. " (Source: mercuryexposure.org. The link to the article no longer works).

Vast research into mercury has shown that it suppresses the immune system and contributes to the development of the viral, fungal and bacterial infections in patients diagnosed with HIV, Herpes Zoster, candidiasis, chronic sinusitis, tonsillitis, bronchitis, kidney, bladder infections, prostatitis, genital herpes, etc. Mercury interferes with the action of antibiotics making them ineffective against bacteria.

Mercury is a silent killer. Since it gets deposited in the nerve tissue, the brain, kidneys, the ganglia and the spinal cord, it is very difficult to diagnose mercury toxicity via routine tests. It does not show in the blood, lymph, urine, faeces, hair. Dr Klinghardt lists four diagnostic procedures which are very complex and some (like the biopsy) are too invasive.

Perhaps the most practical test is the one called the 'challenge' test where complex chelating agents get administered into the body followed by urine analysis. This may be impaired by inadequate levels of calcium sodium and potassium, so these should be raised for the test to give correct information. This test can also be used to analyse the content of other heavy metals in the body.

Cadmium is one of the most toxic metals believed to be more lethal than mercury. Cadmium is one of the most common causes of cancer - more common than any other source. It is a major reason for many other diseases as well, such as cardiovascular, kidney disease, arthritis, diabetes, heart disease. It is also extremely dangerous to a developing foetus since it can easily penetrate the placenta and get into the bloodstream, leading to a development of birth defects and serious conditions for a newly-born child.

Cadmium is found in cigarette smoke, the water we drink and seafood, as well as coffee and tea. Seafood obtained from coastal areas is notorious for cadmium contamination. Junk foods also indirectly affect the levels of cadmium in the body, by being refined, losing important minerals such as zinc, magnesium and calcium in the process.

Cadmium is a known antagonist for zinc. Zinc takes part in the formation of over 100 critical enzymes which are required in cardiovascular, immune, digestive system activity. It is also an antagonist to calcium, manganese, iron, chromium and other useful metals. It raises the sodium levels in the body providing a temporary boost of energy. This is one of the reasons smoking can bring in a sense of well-being and be so addictive.

Psychologically, cadmium is associated with toughness, since it drives copper back into the tissues, calming emotions. Emotional people sometimes resort to smoking to calm their nerves down.

It is also closely associated with mental disorders such as violent, anti-social behaviour, ADHD, etc. Eliminating cadmium by stopping smoking can initially cause a feeling of insecurity and fatigue. However, the feeling passes, and so do violent thoughts.

Arsenic has long been associated with poison. It has been used for political assassinations for many centuries. Arsenic is synonymous with rat poison. It is classified as heavy metal and shares toxic characteristics with other heavy metals such as mercury and lead. Arsenic can be found in contaminated seafood, water supplies, wine and moonshine. It can also be encountered in some herbal preparations.

Poor countries where water supplies and geopolitics are not subject to strict environmental health control are especially at risk from arsenic toxicity. An estimated 100 million people are exposed to heavy metals, including arsenic, from ground and well water. Bangladesh has been named as one of the most exposed nations.

Professor Stephen Marcus, MD, writes: "In Bangladesh, more than 95% of the water supply to over 138 million people is potentially arsenic-contaminated at levels exceeding the US EPA and WHO action limits". He continues in the same article: "Arsenic is listed as a presumed carcinogenic substance based on the increased prevalence of lung and skin cancer observed in human populations with multiple exposures (primarily through industrial inhalation)." (Source: emedicine.com/emerg/topic42.htm)

Non-organic arsenic is more toxic and dangerous that organic. "Trivalent inorganic arsenic inhibits pyruvate dehydrogenase by binding to the sulfhydryl groups of dihydrolipoamide. Consequently, conversion of pyruvate to acetyl coenzyme A (CoA) is decreased, citric acid cycle activity is decreased, and the production of cellular ATP is decreased. Trivalent arsenic inhibits numerous other cellular enzymes through sulfhydryl group binding. Trivalent arsenic inhibits cellular glucose uptake, gluconeogenesis, fatty acid oxidation, and further production of acetyl CoA; it also blocks the production of glutathione, which prevents cellular oxidative damage". (Source: emedicine.com/emerg/topic42.htm)

Lead toxicity – also called saturnism, plumbism, or painter's colic – resulting from an increased level of lead in the body, was first recognized as early as 200 B.C. Nicander of Golopon wrote of lead-induced toxicity characterised by anaemia and colic in 250

B.C. Sugar of lead was used to sweeten wine. This resulted in what is called saturnine gout.

Today most exposure to lead is occupational. It can also be found in leaded paint, petrol, exhaust fumes, some imported cosmetic products, home remedies, toys and other items. Lead-contaminated household dust is cited as the most common reason for lead exposure in children. It mostly comes from leaded paint used to paint the house in the past. In drinking water, lead leaches from lead-containing pipes, faucets and soldier in older buildings. "Other potential sources of lead contamination include brass fixtures, older drinking water coolers, and older coffee urns" (Mushak *et al.* 1989 as cited in AAP 1993). (Source: atsdr.cdc.gov/substances/toxsubstance.asp?toxid=22).

The symptoms of lead poisoning include nausea, abdominal pain, irritability, insomnia, colic, diarrhoea, metal taste, chest pain, colic, etc. Lead can cause irreversible neurological, reproductive damage, as well as renal, cardiovascular and other diseases. Early exposure to lead can also cause severe learning disabilities in children.

Lead toxicity comes from its ability to mimic other metals (e.g. calcium, zinc, iron which play an important role in body processes, such as the formation of enzymes). It replaces these metals, but cannot be utilised as an effective co-factor due to its chemistry.

Aluminium is a trivalent element which is the most abundant metal in the Earth crust. It is one of the elements which have no useful function in the human cell. Aluminium overload and impaired excretion leads to its deposition in the body tissues, such as bones, liver, kidneys, spleen, heart, brain and muscle.

Aluminium enters the body via the gastrointestinal with food, medicines (e.g. aluminium-based antacids) and water. It can also enter the body transdermally from antiperspirants and deodorants. Water presents the highest bioavailability of aluminium via the GI tract.

Aluminium occurs naturally in the drinking water, and acid rain increases its content by releasing it from soils and rocks. Coagulants, such as aluminium sulphate, aluminium chloride and others used in the drinking water treatment increase its concentration even more.

Aluminium toxicity is associated with microcytic anaemia, encephalopathy, and has recently been researched to be connected with Alzheimer's Disease. "Studies show that mice with prolonged exposure to Al soluble salt can develop AD, with selective loss of neurons and the cholinergic function. Al also diminishes the transmission of acetylcholine and attenuates its release, causing reduction of reflexes.

Al appears as a reductor of neuronal activity, showing similarity with the decreased cholinergic action in AD. Al leads to behavioural alterations only in old rabbits, not in the young ones. Thus, mature brains are more susceptible to Al toxicity than immature ones". (Pricilla Costa Ferreira et al, Souce: scielo.br/scielo.php?script=sci_arttext&pid=S0104-11692008000100023&lng=en&nrm=iso&tlng=en)

Aluminium toxicity is usually found in people with impaired renal function. Chronic renal failure may lead to reduced aluminium excretion and its increased concentration in such individuals. "Mechanisms of toxicity include inhibition of enzyme activity and protein synthesis, alterations in nucleic acid function, and changes in cell membrane permeability." (Source: emedicine.medscape.com/article/165315-overview)

7.4. Metabolic Toxins

Metabolic toxins (waste) include the following:

- **Nitrogen waste** – ammonia which forms from the oxidation of amino groups when proteins are converted into carbohydrates. It needs a lot of water to be excreted and is very toxic. The other one is urea, which is less toxic and is also a product of protein metabolism. The third one is uric acid which is the least toxic of them but forms crystals when water is absent.
- **Water and gases** - carbon dioxide, nitrogen, methane.
- **Solids** - these are indigestible parts of food, as well as salts, pigments, dead blood cells, etc. All of these are excreted as faeces.
- When metabolic waste is not cleared up by the body systems timely and efficiently, they become toxic, poisoning the whole body. This can happen due to many factors interfering with the body's ability to eliminate toxic waste:

  - Illness - which can lead to the release of toxins by bacteria, viruses and fungi
  - Not drinking enough water
  - Not sleeping enough
  - Lack of exercise

- Taking recreational drugs
- Certain treatments and medications
- Alcohol abuse (can lead to liver damage)
- Medical conditions which affect organs of elimination (e.g. kidney disease)
- Poisoning due to substance abuse
- Food poisoning
- Toxins formed due to oxidation
- Toxins formed due to stress - acute or chronic.

Symptoms of metabolic toxicity

- Fatigue
- Lack of focus & concentration
- Headaches
- Dizziness
- Nausea
- Vomiting
- Diarrhoea
- Aching muscles & joints
- Infections
- Feeling sleepy & lethargic
- Depression.

7.5. How Toxins Get into the Body

As mentioned earlier, toxins can get into the body with the air, food, water, products we use. They can get into our body via the respiratory tract, digestive system, the skin, mucous membranes of the eyes, mouth, nose and reproductive organs. So what are the sources of modern-day toxins?

Domestic sources:

- Foods: naturally occurring toxins (e.g. mercury in sharks and tuna fish)
- Food additives & dies
- Plastic packaging
- Cooking utensils (e.g. non-stick pans)
- Toiletries (deodorants, shampoos, conditioners, make up)
- Air deodorisers
- Insecticides
- Paints
- Carpets and other floor covering
- PVC
- Toys
- Electronics

- Batteries
- Products of domestic hygiene (chlorine-containing products)
- Some clothes and footwear.

Non-domestic and industrial sources:

- Car fumes
- Pesticides
- Chemical fertilisers
- Industrial waste
- Naturally occurring toxins - UV rays, radon gas, products of volcanic activity, methane gas.
- Industrial accidents which may rupture gas pipes, or create other environmental disasters.
- Natural disasters - volcanic eruptions, tsunamis, tornadoes and hurricanes can damage industrial plants which can result in the release of dangerous toxins.

Other sources:

- Medicines
- Drugs
- Alcohol

- Cigarettes
- Water.

This is not to say that the listed causes and products are toxic and dangerous. The levels of potentially toxic substances are monitored inside the EU, and there are regulations regarding the content of such substances in the EU documents. This is all part of what the environmental protection agencies do.

Nevertheless, it is impossible to monitor and regulate everything. For example, how does one manage smog? Also, the amounts of CO_2 and car exhaust fumes in Central London have on many occasions been reported exceeding permissible levels many times. This creates a lot of challenges in terms of health.

Some toxins we consume willingly - cigarettes, alcohol, drugs. Cigarettes are notorious for their content of heavy metals -, especially cancer-causing cadmium. Medicines and drugs present their challenges. Most medicines have side-effects which can only mean the presence of substances toxic or hazardous to health.

8. The Skin - Its Structure, Functions & Role in Detox

Human Skin

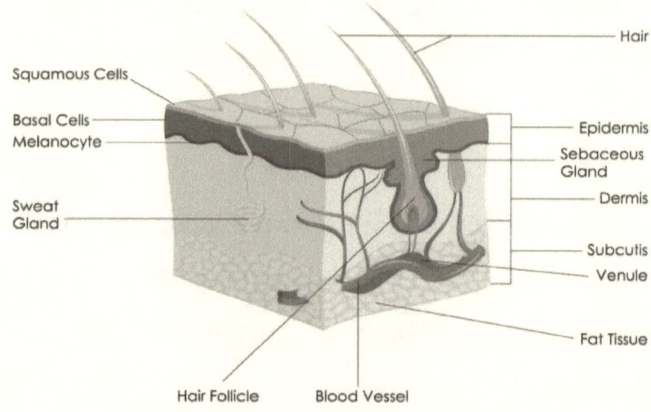

There are seven channels the body uses to get rid of toxins and unwanted matter: the skin, the liver, kidneys, lungs, the intestinal tract, the circulatory and lymphatic systems. They all form the system of elimination. The skin is the largest of them all comprising 12-15% of an adult's body weight. Each square centimetre has 6 million cells, 5,000 sensory points, 100 sweat glands and 15 sebaceous glands.

The skin consists of 3 layers: the epidermis (the outer layer), the dermis ('true skin') and the subcutaneous (fat) layer. Skin is constantly being regenerated. A skin cell starts its life at the lower layer of the skin (the basal layer of the dermis), which is supplied with blood vessels and nerve ending. The cell migrates upward for about two weeks until it reaches the bottom portion of the epidermis, which is the outermost skin layer. The epidermis is not supplied with blood vessels but has nerve endings just like all the other layers.

The skin fulfils 6 very important functions:

1. **Sensation** - the nerve endings in the skin identify touch, heat, cold, pain and light pressure.

2. **Heat regulation** - the skin helps regulate the body temperature by sweating to cool the body down when it overheats and by shivering, creating 'goosebumps' when it is cold. Shivering closes the pores. The tiny hair that stands on end traps warm air and thus helps keep the body warm.

3. **Absorption** - absorption of ultraviolet rays from the sun helps to form vitamin D in the body, which is vital for bone formation. Some creams, essential oils and medicines (e.g. HRT, anti-smoking patches) can also be absorbed through the skin into the bloodstream.

4. **Protection** - the skin protects the body from ultraviolet light - too much of it is harmful to the body - by producing a pigment called melanin. It also protects us from the invasion of bacteria and germs by forming an acid mantle (formed by the skin sebum and sweat). This barrier also prevents moisture loss.

5. **Excretion** - Waste products and toxins are eliminated from the body through the sweat glands. It is a very important function which helps to keep the body 'clean' from the inside.

6. **Secretion** - sebum and sweat are secreted onto the skin surface. The sebum keeps the skin lubricated and soft, and the sweat combines with the sebum to form an acid mantle which creates the right pH balance for the skin to fight off infection.

I would add one more very important but frequently overlooked function to this list – the **diagnostic function**. The skin shows the state of our health. So, when we are ill or otherwise unhealthy, the skin will reflect it immediately. The toxic, congested, tired, stressed body will often have pale, unhealthy complexion. Deprived of proper nourishment and good oxygen supply due to inefficient circulation and elimination, it will be more prone to various skin problems.

It is not only our physical state that affects our skin condition. If a person is affected by continuous psychological stress, the whole body goes into a survival mode, with the endocrine system impacting all the other systems including the skin. Acne, spots, rashes, eczema, dermatitis, psoriasis, ulcers, viral, bacterial and fungal infections are quite common when a person is suffering from physical conditions or psychological stress.

The skin is truly a reflection of our inner health and balance of body and mind. No matter what we do with it to make it more attractive, if we are deprived of health and peace of mind, then any adjustments to our skin will only be superficial, cosmetic and short-lived.

This is why I am sceptical about the effectiveness of a large number of cosmetic products and procedures where the main emphasis is on the skin itself, and not on the state of overall health. If we do not look after our health, such products and procedures are futile and will only drain our wallets and frustrate us with lack of long-term or any visible result. On the other hand, when we look after ourselves by eating the right food, drinking clean water and leading a healthy life, the skin responds by looking healthy and radiant.

Protect it from the environmental damage, exfoliate twice a week, have enough sleep, drink plenty of water, moisturise regularly, use natural masks, massage it occasionally, and the skin will show it is being well looked after. Truly beautiful skin is a result of a life-long effort to maintain a healthy and balanced mind and body.

There are 2 other skin functions the skin has which play a very important role in detoxification and healing: excretion and absorption.

Being the largest organ in the body, the skin can rid the body of a large amount of toxic waste, due to a large number of excretory channels – sweat and sebaceous glands, as well as respiratory channels. Thus it performs the function called *excretion*. The body excretes about 95% of water, with the rest being salts, oil and unwanted substances.

Heavy metals can be successfully excreted with sweat. The skin in this way is a great helper to the body, since many toxins bypass the major organs like the kidneys, colon and liver, reducing any overload and potential damage to them. These organs will themselves need detoxifying if the body is suffering from increased toxicity, so they will not be effective in performing the function of detoxification.

When the body temperature rises, it releases a lot of water in an attempt to cool itself down. This way the skin works like a thermostat for the body fulfilling the function of heat regulation. The higher the temperature, the more we perspire, the more water and salts (including the ones which contain heavy and radioactive metals) we excrete. So, the function of heat regulation is very closely connected to the function of excretion.

Forming a barrier between the body and the environment to protect us from its adverse effects (e.g. water, poisons, bacteria, infections, etc.), the skin can also be highly permeable, especially at raised temperatures, to small water- and oil-soluble molecules and this factor have been increasingly used in medicine to treat a variety of problems. Medicinal patches work thanks to this ability.

Small molecules can penetrate through the skin and enter the circulation. This is the function of the skin called absorption. It works on the same principle as excretion. Since the skin can excrete substances, it can absorb them too, due to its permeability.

With an increase in temperature, the permeability of the skin increases too, so more substances can come in or out of the body. The ability of the skin to speed up excretion and absorption under raised temperatures is widely used in medical, health and beauty treatments. Our ancestors knew that making a sick person sweat helped to expel bad substances, kill germs and speed up recovery. A person would be wrapped up in warm blankets and given plenty of hot sweat-inducing drinks.

Exercise is a great way to get rid of toxins. When we exercise the body gets heated from the inside. To cool itself down, it produces a lot of sweat which escapes through the skin taking water and fat-soluble toxic waste with it.

Another great way to sweat out toxins is in a sauna. Saunas are being used all over the world. Apart from being a wonderfully pleasant experience, it is deeply therapeutic. Regular use of saunas strengthens the heart and blood vessels, stimulates the immune system, relieves any aches and pains in muscles and joints, facilitates the expulsion of toxic waste, including products of metabolic activity and heavy metals, relieves stress, nervous tension, depression, promotes sleep. Regular use of a sauna is one of the best ways to keep the body and mind healthy.

9. Clay-like Minerals

9.1. Zeolite

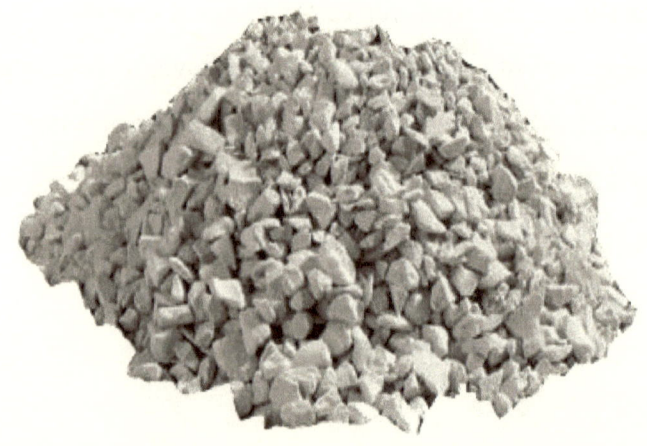

Zeolites are microporous minerals with a well-defined crystalline structure. They belong to a group of natural aluminosilicates. Generally, they contain silicon, aluminium and oxygen in their framework and cations, water and/or other molecules within their pores. The word 'zeolite' consists of two parts: 'zeo' - boil, and 'lithos' - stone ('boiling stones'). This term was originally coined by Axel Fredrick Cronstedt, a Swedish mineralogist in the 18th century. He observed that upon heating a natural mineral rapidly, the stones began to dance about as the water evaporated.

General Information

Zeolites are natural microporous aluminosilicates. which have a crystalline structure and include almost all the chemical elements found in the body. Clinoptilolite is the most abundant member of the 48 minerals in the zeolite group. Its approximate empirical formula is $(Ca, Fe, K, Mg, Na)3-6Si30Al6O72.24H2O$. Typical mineralogical composition: 95% clinoptilolite, minor amounts of feldspar and smectite.

The reason zeolites are now attracting so much interest lies in their strict crystalline structure with minute channels running in different directions which have a negative charge allowing the absorption and adsorption of heavy and radioactive metals and numerous toxins.

Most toxins are positively charged, while zeolites have a negative collective charge, which allows them to act as a sieve for such substances, attracting them into zeolites' numerous channels and removing these toxic substances out of the body. These substances are mostly heavy and radioactive metals.

This property was used during the Chernobyl disaster - a huge amount of zeolite was thrown into the reactors, and was used to de-contaminate people and objects. People were given zeolite with food to help remove radiation out of their bodies. This property is extensively used nowadays by the military forces for the same reasons.

Another very interesting property of zeolites is a selective ionic exchange between the chemical elements in its structure and the environment they are in (e.g. the body of a living organism). Zeolites have almost all the elements of the Periodic Table. Thanks to their ion-exchange property, they provide the body with the elements it needs for healthy functioning while taking out of the body what it has in abundance or simply does not need. This is what can be called an "intelligent" ionic exchange.

In Russia and the United States zeolite (clinoptilolite) is used in the production of food supplements. In some other countries (e.g. Cuba) clinoptilolite has been used to produce an anti-diarrhoea medicine which is successfully used to treat dysentery and other Castro-intestinal disorders, including food poisoning. In Russia clinoptilolite has been included in a group of sorbents. The crystalline structure of zeolites is the only one which cannot be destroyed under any circumstances. It is what is called 'permanently living'.

One more very important factor is the catalytic property of zeolites. It means that they have the potential to normalise biochemical processes in the body which cannot take place without certain micro- and macro-elements. These elements are supplied to the body by zeolites.

Zeolite and Animals

Zeolites are the most accessible minerals to both animals and humans. Animals have been observed to restore their mineral homoeostasis by gorging on natural zeolites (up to 10-20kg!). There is a name for this phenomenon - lithophagia. Nowadays zeolites are used in agriculture in Russia in animal feeds to strengthen the immune system of farm animals, regulate metabolism and prevent Castro-intestinal infection. The result is healthy offspring, healthy growth and good overall health. They have also demonstrated increased fertility and the birth of healthy offspring in a large number of studies on animals.

Zeolites have a strictly calibrated pore size (about 4 Angstroms - A). This allows a zeolite structure to be absorbent only concerning ions of micro- and macro-elements and structures of small sizes (ammonia, hydrogen sulphate, methane, etc., without getting in direct contact with vitamins, amino acids, proteins and other complex organic structures). This means that compared to other sorbents which should not normally be taken longer than 2 weeks, clinoptilolite can be used for a long time, since it does not absorb (and consequently does not extract) the above mentioned important substances (vitamins, amino acids, proteins, etc.) out of the body. Zeolite simply cannot absorb them due to a small structure of its channels.

Properties

- Very strong "magnet" for heavy and radioactive metals. This property is used where exposure to radiation is a risk.
- Acts as a sponge for toxins.
- Promotes the removal of free radicals.

Uses and applications

Like clays, zeolite is used in baths, poultices, body wraps, beauty treatments – such as scrubs, exfoliators, face masks, beauty wraps.

Bath

For a bath 300g of zeolite is normally used, mixed with very warm water. The water needs to be stirred occasionally to promote the process of detoxification. Some sea salt (about 300g) can be added to the bath to increase the potency. However, care regarding salt needs to be taken if suffering from high blood pressure, heart conditions or any other health problems.

Poultice

For a poultice, zeolite can be mixed with warm water to a fairly thick paste to be applied in a thick layer on aching muscles, joints, bruises, etc., for 1-2 hours at a time.

Compress

Same as a poultice, only a more liquid consistency, laid on a piece of cloth and applied for 1 hour. Wrap the area with cling film and a warm scarf for better effect.

Wrap

A wrap is a potent treatment. Zeolite can be an addition to a clay or seaweed wrap, to promote toxin removal through the skin. It can be mixed with clay or seaweed in a 1:1 consistency.

9.2. Diatomaceous Earth

Diatomaceous Earth (DE, diatomite, kieselguhr) is a naturally occurring, soft, chalk-like, sedimentary rock mineral that is easily crumbled into a fine white or beige powder. This powder is very light-weight due to its high porosity. It is made primarily of silica and consists of fossilized remains of diatoms - hard-shelled algae which inhabited the waters of the Earth millions of years ago.

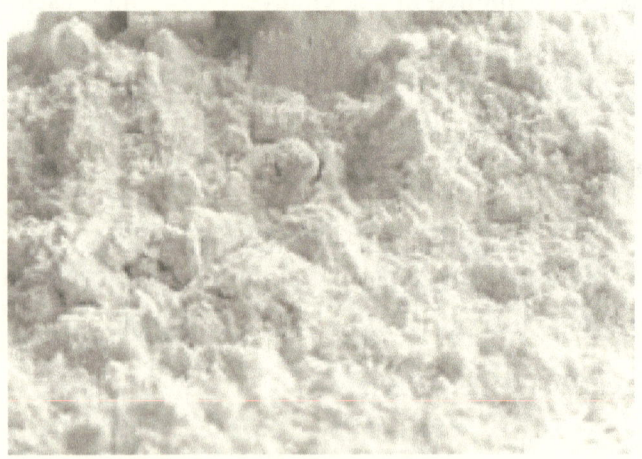

Diatoms used to serve as the basic food for aquatic life, just as grass is the basic food for land animals. Some of these deposits which gradually shifted to the dry land are extremely important to humans.

There are hundreds of sources of Diatomaceous Earth and most deposits are from saltwater sources. DE coming from freshwater sources is of extremely high purity and is therefore called food-grade diatomite. Freshwater diatomite is mined from dry lake beds and is mostly hydrated amorphous silica.

Food grade DE is non-toxic and is safe around humans, animals, pets, plants and the environment. Its 100% natural origin ensures that it is free from artificial chemicals which are abundant in modern-day insecticides, anti-parasite remedies and plant food.

How does it work on insects/parasites?

Diatomite punctures the exoskeleton of insects and parasites and absorbs their body fluids, effectively drying them out. It also acts as a powerful natural repellent. Insects stay away from surfaces covered with DE, making a serious infestation unlikely. When ingested, it destroys parasites by puncturing their skin and absorbing fluids. It makes food-grade DE the most powerful and safe natural insecticide/anti-parasite natural remedy around.

Uses of Diatomaceous Earth

At home

Use against house insects (ants, cockroaches, silverfish, bed bugs, flies, fleas, box elder bugs, scorpions, crickets, ticks, etc.). Sprinkle the areas which you suspect is infested with insects. To eliminate bed bugs, sprinkle it over the bed generously.

Pet protection against insects and parasites - fleas, ticks, lice, and other pests. Rub the powder into the animal fur, sprinkle on the carpet, bedding. Against parasites - add 0.5-1 tsp of DE to pet food or water to expel parasites and prevent their re-appearance. Cat litter - add for odour control.

Livestock protection against insects and parasites

Horses, cows, pigs, sheep, goats, rabbits, chickens, and other domestic animals will benefit from the use of DE to protect them against fly larvae, ticks, fleas, etc. Add DE to animal feed to expel parasites.

Livestock - other benefits

Regular addition of DE to animal feed will stimulate metabolic rate, improve coat and hoof condition, improve digestion and elimination, act as a natural mineral food supplement (it contains numerous minerals in it), promote healthier egg production and stronger eggs in poultry, and reduce overall animal stress. It will also reduce the odour in barns from excrement, prevent larvae from forming in the manure. All of this will help reduce vet bills.

For smaller farm animals (pigs, sheep, goats), add about 12g (0.5oz) to their feed. For larger animals (cows, horses), add 25-50g of DE to feed, once a day. For poultry and small animals which you keep in large number add 2% of DE to their food.

Natural plant protection against insects

DE is the organic way of controlling insects in the garden, greenhouse, orchard, and more. Use it for control of slugs, whitefly, beetles, mites, grasshoppers, etc. For use in the greenhouse or outdoors on fruits, vegetables, flowers, grains and grass - up to and including the day of harvest. Ensure coverage over the entire plant, including under the leaves. For young plants, two pounds per acre may be adequate.

For larger plants, five lb/acre may be enough. Examine the leaves periodically to make sure that the DE goes all over the plant and the leaves are not eaten by bugs. Use special dust applicator. Make sure that you always wear a protective mask over the face and your eyes are covered to avoid irritation of the eyes/mucous membrane.

Can DE be used by humans?

I believe it can be. Food grade diatomaceous earth is used to protect grains from infestation. Many people swear by it for getting rid of parasites (intestinal worms). With all this, I have heard a lot of anecdotal evidence of blood sugar level normalising, condition of the skin, hair and nails improving. Some people have reported a reduction in appetite and weight loss. Latin American DE is good and very pure, consisting almost of 100% amorphous silica. Question your sources when purchasing DE if you consider taking it internally.

10. Mud

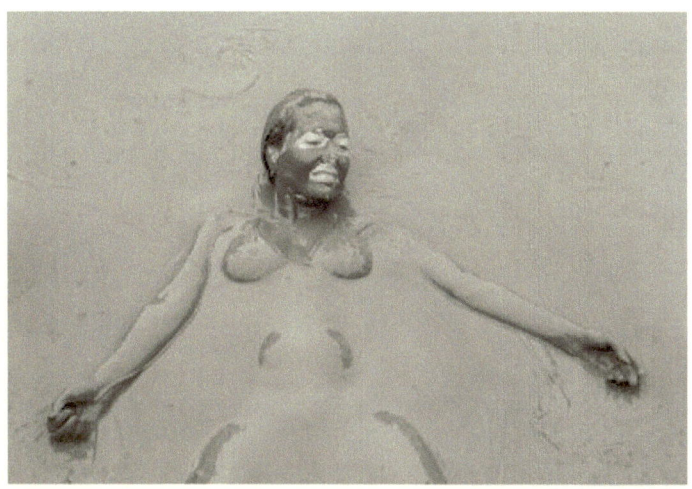

Muds, otherwise known as peloids, have been used by people and animals for thousands of years. We all know about the urge of many animals to cover themselves in mud - for a variety of reasons known only to them. They are instinctively drawn to mud - they roll in it, they eat it... Humans have also been using mud since times immemorial. There is no arguing about the fact that mud is good for us. It is extremely rich both in minerals and organic substances which have been used in peloid therapy for centuries, bringing incredible results.

A great number of resorts all over the world using muds for treatment of various health conditions and health maintenance, as well as spas and beauty salons where muds are used to improve skin condition and for weight management, proves the fact that mud works. The use of muds as a therapeutic substance is based on their ability to stimulate metabolism and their analgesic, anti-inflammatory and adaptogenic qualities.

If we also consider the fact that the popularity of muds has grown immensely in the past few years and is on a steady increase, then one can explain the fact that people want to know more about muds and how they work on the body.

There are different types of mud. We know of moor mud, salt lake mud, sea mud and other types. For many years cosmetic manufacturers have researched various muds from across the globe analysing their healing components and have incorporated them into their skincare and body care product lines. Today we come across anything from mud masks and mud soaps to mud creams both in spas and available to us from retail shops.

10.1. What Are Muds?

Muds consist of humus and minerals. They are formed over a very long time by physical, chemical, biological and geological processes. The original material for mud formation is algae, plants, crustaceans and other substances. As a result of biochemical processes, the decomposition of organic matter in muds has led to the formation in them of amino acids, salts of fatty acids, aroma-substances, etc. The most mobile matter in mud consists of fatty acids, carbohydrates and amino acids. These organic compounds are important for life activity of the microflora in muds - they keep them "alive".

As a result of biochemical processes, in the presence of bacteria, complex organic compounds are formed, such as humic acids, fulvic acids, antioxidants, and many other substances. Structurally, muds represent a complex physicochemical system which consists of 3 interconnected parts: liquid (the mud solution), the solid matter, and the colloidal complex.

When it comes from saltwater sources, the mud solution consists of water and salts dissolved in it. It is the derivative of brine ("rapah") - a water solution with a high concentration of salts which covers mud deposits. The concentration of salts in the mud solution can vary drastically - from 0.01g/l in moor peats and sapropels, to 350g/l in sulphide silts. Within the same deposit, the concentration of the solution can vary considerably - up to 5 times, depending on the season and hydro-meteorological changes.

The solid matter consists of particles of various origin - salt and mineral crystals and rough organic matter. They are over 0.001mm in diameter. The higher peloids are in Small particles, the higher their plasticity, and the better their quality from the therapeutic point of view. The presence of particles over 0.25mm in diameter should not exceed 2-3% for therapeutic peloids.

Colloidal complex - finely dispersed component of muds - consists of various mineral particles below 0.001mm in diameter and presents a plastic hydrophilic basis which determines water saturation capacity and heat retention capability of mud. The colloidal content differs depending on the type of mud. In silts, it is 4-20%, in moor peats and sapropels (with a high content of organic matter), it reaches up to 80%.

The main mud groups are:

- Low moor peats
- High moor peats
- Sapropel muds
- Sulphide silt muds

Moor peats (low and high) are also referred to as organic mud (or torf). This type of mud has been formed as a result of partial bacterial decomposition of micro- and macro- vegetation in conditions of high humidity and low oxygenation. It normally contains more than 50% of organic matter, with the degree of bacterial decomposition of 40% or more. Moor peats are normally very rich in the humic matter (up to 47% in dry matter).

Sapropel muds are silts of freshwater origin. They are rich in organic matter (more than 10%) and are formed as a result of multiple macro- and microbiological 7processing of water plants and animals. Unlike moor peats, sapropels are not as rich in the humic matter (20-25% of dry matter).

Sulphide silt muds are of saltwater origin. They are relatively poor in organic matter (less than 10%) and, as a rule, are rich in iron sulphide (FeS) and water-soluble salts. They can be subdivided into low-sulphide (FeS content of 0.01-0.15%), medium-sulphide (0.15-0.5%), and high-sulphide (over 0.5%) silts.

As far as mineral content is concerned, therapeutic muds are also subdivided into fresh-water muds (ash/mineral content of mud solution of up to 1g/litre), muds with low mineral content (1-15 g/l), muds with medium mineral content (15-35g/l), high mineral content muds (35-150g/l), saturated muds (150-300g/l), and over-saturated muds (over 300g/l).

Acidity also varies - from ultra-acidic (with pH of 1.5-2, as in organic moor peats), to alkaline (pH over 9, as in sulphide silt muds).

The most frequently used in therapeutic practice are sulphide silt muds, followed by sapropels. This may be explained, on the one hand, by their abundance, and on the other hand - by extensive research data on them.

10.2. How Do Muds Work?

The action of muds on the body systems is a combination of the temperature (heat), mechanical and chemical factors.

The temperature (or heat) factor is considered by some to be the most important physical factor in peloid therapy. It has been established that heat increases the activity of chemical components in peloids. Besides, heated mud promotes swelling of the skin which changes penetrability of cellular membranes for biochemically active components of muds.

According to the "chemical" theory, chemically active substances found in peloids (hormones, antibiotics, bio stimulators, microelements, organic acids) penetrate the body systems and heal the body from the inside. Heat and other physical factors, in this case, are deemed as a subsidiary, based on tests in which peloids were applied at hot and cold temperatures.

The fact that peloid molecules can penetrate through the skin into the body has been proved by scientists a few decades ago. Hydrogen sulphate is considered a biologically active component of muds. It acts in a way similar to acetylcholine, causing substantial changes in the circulatory system. It raises blood pressure, slows down the pulse and narrows blood vessels, thus changing the blood supply to organs and body tissues and improving the heart activity.

Bio-stimulating effect of muds has been connected by some scientists with their antioxidant properties which most of them possess. Because of the way mud works on the circulatory system, it should be used with great caution by people who have cardiac disease and blood pressure problems. Clay does not have the same effect, which makes it a safer choice for people with cardiac and blood pressure problems.

In 1973, P.G.Tsarfis offered a theory according to which peloid application increases penetrability of the skin to their components, and in particular, to iron. Iron and other elements of peloids penetrate from the surface of the skin deep into the body systems.

An increase of biochemical enzyme activity on the cellular and sub-cellular levels takes place, which leads to an appearance of a "centre of pathology" where one can observe changes in the levels of biologically active substances, an increase in the content of acid mucopolysaccharides, heparin, with the content of hyaluronic acids remaining unchanged.

These local changes initiate regional and reflex processes, with the participation of the central nervous system which regulates the release of biologically active substances, neurohormones, thus intensifying enzyme-releasing systems. Integrative and neuro-humoral processes act selectively, first of all - on the most reactive systems, i.e. systems affected by pathology, since they are the least resistant.

Compensatory mechanisms are switched on, on various levels, through the peripheral nerve formations. As a result of all this, the following takes place: an increase in hormonal activity and intracellular steroidal metabolic activity, a reduction in tissue penetrability, as well as inflammatory components and autoimmune aggression, and slowing down of collagen destruction.

It is important to remember that reaction to a mud procedure depends on the condition of the body systems and the intensity of therapeutic factors. As a result of many years of research, it has been established that at the basis of peloid therapy is its ability to normalise of the body, tissues and cells.

It is important to note that muds have different combinations of biologically active substances which make them differ in their clinical effectiveness. They affect different regulatory and homoeostatic body systems. Such selective effect of muds is explained by the fact that, first of all, like different oil deposits, each of them is formed only in certain regions of our planet in unique geological conditions, and secondly, each type of mud has an age, being at a certain stage of ethnogenesis (or maturity). At the basis of this process lies the activity of a whole group of micro-organisms, with the products of their activity forming the basis of therapeutic properties of muds.

V.I.Vernadskiy has called mud "the living matter" of our planet which reflects the processes of its evolution and regional geochemical specifics. Considering this, there is an opinion that there are "old" and "new" muds, differing from each other in the combination of biologically active substances, as well as their biological, clinical and sanogenetic effects.

By stimulating systemic restructuring of the antioxidant status of the organism and changing the structure of the neuroendocrine and immune regulatory functions, natural peloids activate reparative reactions in the body. As well as antioxidant properties, mud also has analgesic and anti-inflammatory effect, boosting the immune system and acting as adaptogens.

Antioxidant properties of muds are based on the presence of carotene and its analogues (discovered by the spectral analysis). This makes muds effective at treating many diseases of an inflammatory nature, since antioxidants, and particularly carotene, regulate physicochemical characteristics of body membranes.

In recent years, carotenoids, and in particular, beta-carotene, has been successfully used as a preventative treatment for tumours, IBS, to correct unfavourable effects of the environment on the human organism, since they stimulate protective functions of the body systems and activate humoral and cellular immunity.

Retinoids are another group of antioxidants present in mud which possess immune-boosting functions. It is possible that due to their anti-oxidant function, retinoids can actively promote micro-circulation. Also, a comparative analysis of muds and moor peats has shown that antioxidant properties of mud are more prominent than those of peats.

Based on research conducted by Siberian scientists, the following **conclusions** can be made:

1. Therapeutic and adaptogenic properties of muds are both directly targeted at the areas of pathology and indirectly affect endocrine glands, and particularly adrenal glands.

2. Biologically active compounds in muds can sufficiently influence the activity of the endocrine glands as a result of a targeted action comparable to the one in anti-oxidant therapy.

3. Based on their physicochemical characteristics, muds are widely used to treat a large number of conditions of musculoskeletal, genitourinary, digestive, nervous, integumentary (skin), endocrine (hormones), respiratory, circulatory and lymphatic systems.

4. Although a mud-based treatment does cause a balneological reaction ("healing crisis"), their action on the body is mostly mild and is targeted not only at the area of pathology but at all the body systems.

5. The ultimate goal of peloid therapy is to rebalance the body systems and restore homoeostasis.

The main therapeutic properties of muds which are used in peloid therapy are:

1. Powerful antioxidant
2. Peptide
3. Anti-ageing
4. Anti-inflammatory
5. General healing.

10.3. Dead Sea Mud

One of the best-known muds in the world comes from the Dead Sea. Dead Sea Mud is black and enriched with such healing minerals as magnesium, calcium, potassium, bromide, and organic remains of plants and animals. It is the organic matter in mud which makes it such a potent healing and beauty product.

Dead Sea mud has long been known for its therapeutic properties. It has been used to treat conditions such as arthritis, rheumatism, body aches and pains, eczema, psoriasis, acne, inflammations, infertility, and many others. It contains a high concentration of salts and minerals, forming a unique combination not found in any other body of water in the world.

10.4. What is the Difference between Mud & Clay?

Although in some countries (e.g. USA) the word "mud" implies both mud and clay, strictly speaking, clay is very different from the mud. Mud has been formed as a result of deposition over a very long time (sometimes millions of years) of dead trees, plants, animals and insects. This is why it is so rich in organic matter. Clay is formed as a result of deposition of volcanic ash which is inorganic in origin. This is why clay consists mostly of minerals rather than organic matter.

Properties of clay and mud are different too. Mud is usually a very active substance, while the clay is a lot softer in its action on the body. The other thing is - mud should not be taken internally. Many clays, on the other hand, can be ingested safely.

10.5. Uses & Applications

Application methods for mud are the same as for clays – compress, poultice, bath, face mask, body wrap, body mask, as cosmetic ingredients, or a medium for balneological procedures.

Muds are traditionally used by medical spas to treat the following medical conditions:

- Arthritis and rheumatism
- Eczema
- Psoriasis
- Acne
- Fertility problems
- Stress-related disorders
- Poor circulation
- Fatigue

- Poor immunity
- Respiratory problems
- Disorders of the Nervous System.

11. Therapeutic & Beauty Applications of Clays

11.1. Clay Baths

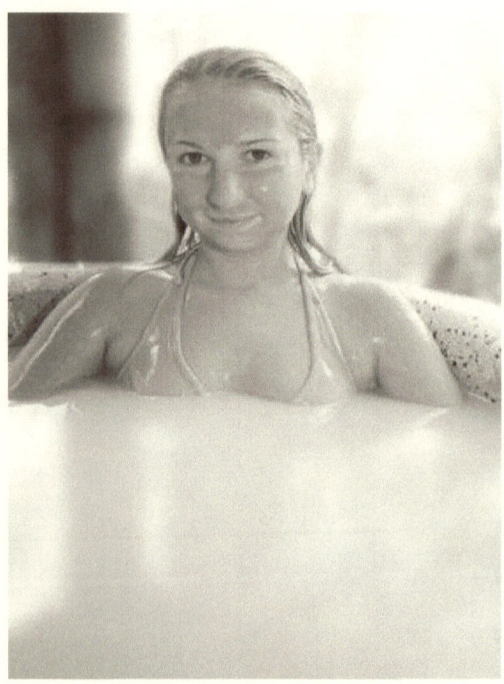

Detoxifying and therapeutic effects of clays are best experienced when used in a bath. Raised body temperatures widen the pores and speed up blood circulation and lymphatic drainage. More toxins are delivered to and can be excreted by the skin than at normal temperatures.

Raised temperatures also speed up healing processes in the body, since all body reactions happen many times faster. Clays absorb these toxins in large quantities while providing the body with essential minerals. This makes the process of detoxification much more profound.

Jason Eyton, researcher and founder of what in my view is the best non-commercial website about clays for medicinal purposes, of eytonsearth.org, cites Dr Miriam Jang, MD who has researched autism and efficacy of various detoxifying substances to reduce heavy metal toxicity:

"...I have put a huge number of patients on these clay baths and the levels of heavy metals – mercury, lead, arsenic, aluminium, and cadmium have come down dramatically...I have been monitoring the levels of metals using all three methods (TD DMPS, oral DMSA and clay baths)and the clay baths are way faster in the removal of metals..."

..."One particular patient had very high levels of mercury and levels of lead that were off the charts. In 3 months of twice-weekly clay baths, the lead came down dramatically and the mercury disappeared. The muscle weakness associated with high lead levels improved dramatically. Interestingly enough, another 5 months of these clay baths showed even lower levels of lead but the mercury reappeared. This supports the theory that mercury is sequestered in different areas of our body and it takes time to get it all out." - Dr Miriam Jang, M.D. , author of "Breakthroughs in Autism", a synopsis of the DAN protocol. (Source: miriamjangmd.com/bio.html)

The most suitable clays for detoxification procedures are calcium and sodium bentonite and variations of these, green montmorillonite and illite, blue Cambrian clay, Fuller's earth, Canadian glacial clay, and many others.

Muds and salts can be added to clay baths as a source of extra minerals, peptides, amino-acids, anti-oxidants and other biologically active substances. These facilitate detoxification and support the mineral balance of the body. Note, however, that muds are more biologically active than clays, due to a high presence of organic substances, so they should be used with caution by people with suspected tumours, heart problems, abnormal blood pressure, epilepsy, acute and severe health conditions. If in doubt, avoid mud.

How much clay should you use per bath? The more clay is used - the better. However, for most people, it may not be the answer, since clays do cost money, and if they have to be transported, then the expense can be high. Two to three kilograms of dry clay would make a good effective detoxifying bath, but half a kilo can be sufficient too.

How much water should be used? You need enough to submerge the whole body. The water temperature should on average be higher than the body temperature – about 40-42°C. However, if it feels uncomfortable, make it cooler.

Having one bath a week is a great way to start. This can be increased to 2-3 times a week. Adding Epsom salt or magnesium chloride to the bath will make it more effective.

11.2. Clay Masks

Clays are a wonderful and very traditional medium for face masks. They have been used in beauty rituals since prehistoric times. There are records of clay being used by ancient Egyptians, the Chinese, the Romans and the Aztecs. The great advantage of clay is that it is powerful as it is, mixed with water – without the addition of extra ingredients. However, ingredients are added to enhance multiple properties of clays.

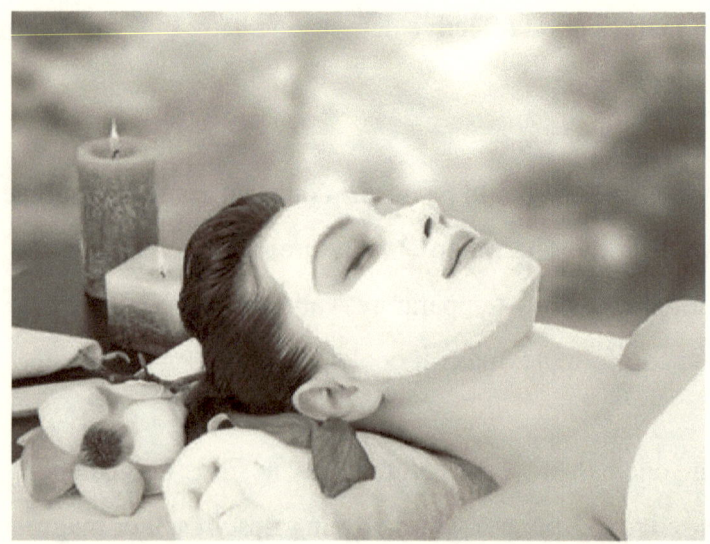

Following are ideas for mask recipes using various clays available in nature.

Acne, oily skin

Green illite is one of the best clays to deal with acne and oily skin, due to its great ability to absorb, apart from its natural disinfectant properties. The clay should be mixed with warm water into a smooth runny paste and applied on the skin as a mask, for 10-15 minutes. Wash off when it dries up, tone with a freshly-made cucumber juice, and apply jojoba or coconut oil to soften and condition the skin afterwards. Jojoba oil is great for oily skin since it has the same pH as the skin, so has a protective action.

Broken capillaries

Mix red Illite clay with rose water to a paste. Apply on the skin as required, let dry, remove and apply toner and moisturiser suitable for your skin type.

Ageing skin (dry, sensitive)

Face mask for dry ageing skin - mix 2 tbsp of pink illite clay with rose water and 3 drops of rose essential oil.

Ageing skin (oily)

For oily ageing skin mix equal parts of yellow illite with water and freshly squeezed cucumber juice. Squeeze some lemon. Apply, leave to dry and wash off. Apply a toner and moisturiser after the mask has been washed off.

11.3. Clay Wraps

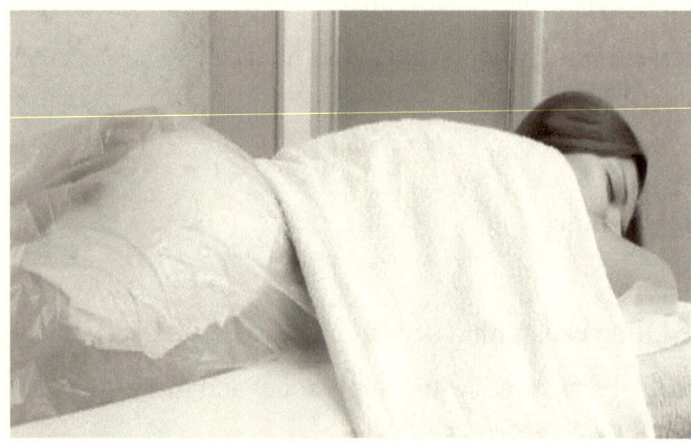

A body wrap is a luxurious and thoroughly therapeutic treatment. It works wonders not only on the skin but on the whole body, due to the ability of the skin to absorb and excrete.

Wraps can be straightforward, by simply using a product and wrapping materials. They can also be thermal, which makes the product work faster and on a deeper level.

Clays, alongside muds, are some of the most popular products in body wraps, due to their own very potent properties – to draw toxins, remineralise and heal. Here are just some of the uses of clay in body wraps:

- Detoxification
- Weight loss
- Rejuvenation
- Skin problems
- Aches & pains
- General healing
- pH balance.

Similar to masks, certain types of clays can be used depending on the type of skin and the goal of treatment.

- Green illite clay is great for oily, acne-prone skin.
- Green montmorillonite, calcium bentonite and Canadian Glacial clay are great for detox and weight loss.
- Sodium bentonite is excellent for acidic conditions, due to its high alkalinity.
- Red illite clay is a great choice for ageing sallow skin.
- Pink illite clay is soft, mildly absorbing clay – great for sensitive problem skin.
- Yellow illite clay is a fantastic choice for any type of skin. It is mild, so can be very beneficial for ageing problem skin.

- Blue Cambrian clay is very potent in detoxification procedures.

You may have to do several treatments on a client to find out which clay their body responds best to. With time you will learn to be intuitive and will be choosing the clay which is most appropriate for the type of skin and goals you are pursuing. We will talk more about wraps a bit later.

11.4. Far Infrared Sauna

Far infrared technology is a relatively recent invention. It is based on the use of infrared heating devices which allow deep penetration of radiant heat into the body at about half the temperature created by conventional saunas (110-120°F against 180-220°F). There are variations of far infrared devices, such as a wooden sauna and a bag/wrap, with the second one being more suitable for home use.

When exposed to far-infrared procedures, the skin is warmed up gradually and deeply. It is accompanied by the dilation of blood vessels, stimulation of sweat and sebaceous glands followed by profound sweating and excretion of sebum. With sweat and oil, the skin can expel a considerable amount of toxins – both organic and inorganic.

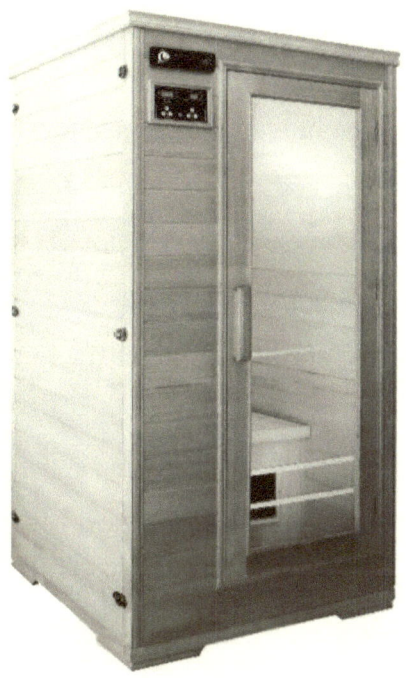

The toxins we accumulate contain heavy metals, and making the body sweat deals causes them to be excreted via the skin, bypassing the liver, intestinal tract and kidneys, which eases the load on these vital organs. It is passive, but very effective detoxification.

Thus, far infrared sauna has the following therapeutic effects:

- It speeds up circulation bringing more nutrients and oxygen to the body organs and the skin and removing a large amount of toxic waste.
- It speeds up body metabolism.
- It increases the production of red and white blood cells.
- The increase in body temperature helps to relax the muscles and other body tissues, thus bringing relief of muscle and joint aches and pains.
- The dilation of the blood vessels promotes the reduction in the diastolic blood pressure.
- It has anti-bacterial, anti-viral and anti-fungal action by reducing the infection due to raised body temperature (the 'fever' effect).
- It exercises the heart muscle.
- It improves peripheral circulation.
- It has a calming effect on the central nervous system.
- It improves immunity thus helping to fight infection.

A far infrared sauna bag is the most convenient one for home detox and treatments.

11.5. Doing a Far Infrared Clay Wrap at Home

To do a clay wrap at home, you will need a plastic sheet and a far infrared sauna set on a moderate setting. It can be an electric blanket, but the effect will not be the same as from a far infrared device. You will also need a warm room and someone to apply clay on for you if you find it difficult to do it yourself. If you suffer from heart problems, blood pressure abnormalities, circulation disorders, thermal clay wraps may not be the right thing for you, so consult with your doctor.

Prepare everything for the wraps. You will need clay, warm water, salt (magnesium chloride is the best one), a thin plastic sheet the size of your body (to wrap yourself in) and a warm blanket. An electric blanket or an infrared sauna blanket – both on a moderate setting – will boost the effect from the treatment. For the first time use any warming devices on a low setting. You need to get used to the clay and take note of how it works with your body. Moderation is essential for any long-term stable results.

Once the clay has been mixed with water (add some magnesium chloride-based salt – either flakes mixed with water – 1table spoonful (tbsp) per 200ml of water, or magnesium oil – 1-2 tbsp per application), apply either on the whole body or on the parts needing attention – similar to a poultice/compress application.

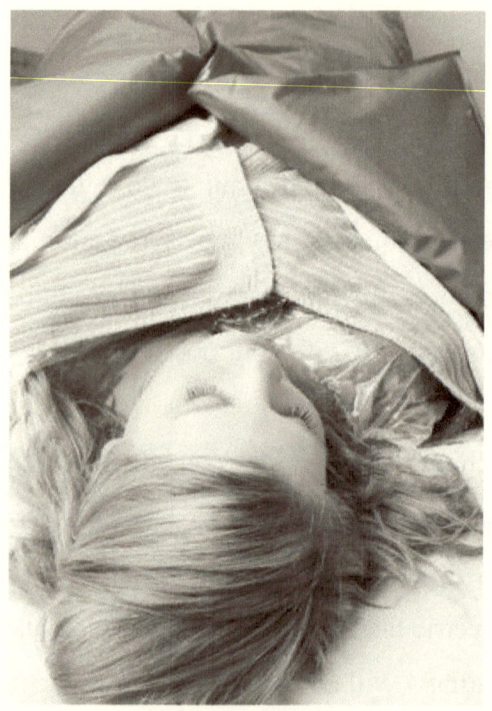

Spread the product all over the body or the area you would like to treat, wrap yourself with a plastic sheet and warm blanket. An electric blanket or far-infrared sauna can be used at low-temperature settings.

It is important to keep yourself warm. The duration of the procedure will vary from 40 minutes to an hour. Warm applications are contra-indicated in cases of inflammations or acute conditions. Where there is excessive heat generated in the body (normally a result of inflammations), cold is appropriate. In such cases, a normal poultice/compress application will be sufficient.

And the other way round is also true – if a condition is associated with cold, energy and organ deficiency, then warm temperatures should be used. This principle has been observed for thousands of years in Traditional Chinese medicine and has been proved to work.

As a general rule, remember that clays are active substances, and one needs to try them out at a body temperature first, raising it gradually to a level which can be comfortably tolerated.

Proper and timely hydration is essential, so drink plenty of water before, during and after the procedure. A bit of Himalayan salt can be added to the water if you are sweating a lot. A cup of herbal tea – e.g. peppermint with dandelion root, or milk thistle, with added honey, or honey and lemon, or just simple lemon water - can be taken instead of pure water. These drinks will stimulate detoxification of the liver and through it of the entire body.

Magnesium chloride, Epsom or Himalayan salt can be added to the clay preparation. Salts will stimulate the system and remineralise the body through the skin. Magnesium chloride and magnesium chloride-containing salts will help to ease aches and pains, relax muscles, soothe joints, promote detoxification, blood circulation and healthy skin, reduce anxiety and nervous tension. Himalayan salt will help to remineralise the body and raise its temperature, promoting sweating and weight loss.

11.6. Doing a Far Infrared Clay Wrap in a Clinic

Clay wraps are a great way to treat patients for many physical conditions. In beauty clinics, clay wraps can be used to promote detoxification and weight loss, as well as skin rejuvenation.

Application procedures are similar to the ones in home conditions. For health problems, clay should be mixed with warm water into a paste (preferably filtered tap water if natural spring water is unavailable). Warm seawater can be a good alternative. However, it makes a clay mixture more active and stimulating, so care needs to be taken where stimulation is contraindicated.

Sodium chloride and sea salt (which is high in sodium chloride) are stimulating. Magnesium chloride-based salts, on the other hand, are relaxing, physically and mentally, so have no such contra-indications and add to the numerous therapeutic benefits of clays.

Having been mixed with water, clay paste needs some warming up on a water bath, to the desired temperature. Most body wraps need to be warmer than the normal body temperature, but not hot. The temperature can be increased gradually for the follow-up procedures to a higher setting.

As I have mentioned above, the whole body coverage is not always essential or appropriate, and sometimes only the part or parts which need attention can be treated. Remember that the deeper the problem (e.g. liver needing detoxification), the thicker should be the layer of clay spread over the area. The application should be wider than the treated area, since surrounding tissues may be affected as well, so make sure that the coverage spreads by about 5cm beyond the area being treated.

It is not always advisable to use heat with clay wraps. Sometimes a cold clay compress is more appropriate. For example, in cases of inflammations or acute recent injuries (e.g. contusion, muscle, joint, tendon, or ligament injury) heat is contra-indicated. The rule is – if an area is hot, or red, or characterised by recent bruising, or sharp pain – use cold clay applications.

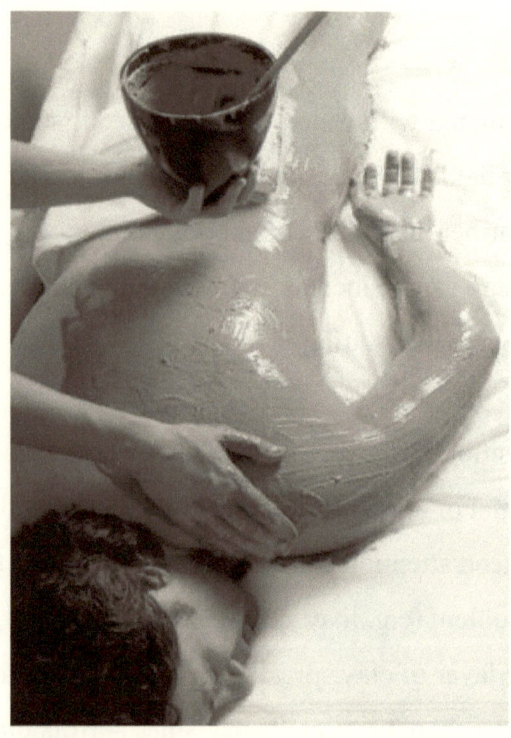

A contusion, strain or sprain, for example, can often lead to bleeding within the body tissues (manifested as bruising). A cold compress or poultice will reduce the bleeding and help prevent inflammation, as well as the duration of an injury. Such applications need to be applied frequently (once every 1-2 hours or so) following an injury. Ice may be used in conjunction with the procedures.

As the area starts healing (normally on the 3rd day from the moment of injury), warm applications, together with massage procedures will facilitate healing processes in the area. Warm clay and massage will stop tissues from sticking together and forming lumps. Such lumps are a common cause of secondary injuries in the area, as well as chronic pain and tension.

Dr Vesna Humo, who is a surgeon, has all her patients use clay after mastectomy with radiotherapy. She advises patients to use clay directly on the skin to prevent skin damage and has seen excellent results from this. Importantly she is using clay for bed sores and every necrotic and septic wound also with excellent results. In addition to clay and saunas, which have both been used since the dawn of civilization, we now have new emerging technologies that also use the skin as avenues of toxic escape.

To learn about how to do the treatments using minerals and far-infrared on yourself and your clients, please refer to the links at the end of this book.

12. A Word of Caution

I hope that after reading this book you have learned a bit more about clays, muds and clay-like minerals and why they work with our body the way they do.

The main thing to remember is that clays and clay-like minerals are not drugs, and should never be used to replace medical treatment. They work with the body holistically, and not as medicines.

If you have any health problems which have not been diagnosed yet, make sure that you seek medical advice.

If you are on medication or are undergoing treatment, ask your GP for advice on whether the products or treatments described in this book are safe for you to use.

Further Information & Links

Other books from the Mineral Healing series:

amazon.com/author/galinastgeorge

Email:

support@purenaturecures.com

Website:

Purenaturecures.com

www.ingramcontent.com/pod-product-compliance
Lightning Source LLC
Chambersburg PA
CBHW050447290526
45786CB00006B/2194